Environmental Health Noncompliance

Environmental Health Noncompliance

A Sanitarian's Search for a New System

David Mikkola, R.S., M.P.H.

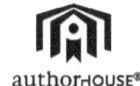
authorHOUSE®

AuthorHouse™
1663 Liberty Drive
Bloomington, IN 47403
www.authorhouse.com
Phone: 1-800-839-8640

© 2013 by David Mikkola, R.S., M.P.H.. All rights reserved.

No part of this book may be reproduced, stored in a retrieval system, or transmitted by any means without the written permission of the author.

Published by AuthorHouse   04/09/2013

ISBN: 978-1-4817-3682-4 (sc)
ISBN: 978-1-4817-3705-0 (hc)
ISBN: 978-1-4817-3706-7 (e)

Library of Congress Control Number: 2013906314

Any people depicted in stock imagery provided by Thinkstock are models, and such images are being used for illustrative purposes only.
Certain stock imagery © Thinkstock.

This book is printed on acid-free paper.

Because of the dynamic nature of the Internet, any web addresses or links contained in this book may have changed since publication and may no longer be valid. The views expressed in this work are solely those of the author and do not necessarily reflect the views of the publisher, and the publisher hereby disclaims any responsibility for them.

CONTENTS

The Inspection-Based Enforcement Approach to Noncompliance 1
Support for the Inspection System 4
A Critique of the System 9
Considering Objections to Change 10
The Profession's Development and Mindset 12
Over Emphasis on Legal Enforcement 20
Effects of Fear Arousal and Anxiety 23
Fear Arousal Summary 34
Critique: Poor Design of Education and Communication Efforts 36
Considering a New Paradigm 45
Section Summary: Learning Principles 51
The Health Belief Model 52
Implementing Changes: Introduction to Intervention Design 79
Designing the Intervention 81
Using the Model During Intervention Design 86
Making a Persuasive Argument for Change 90
Actual Versus Perceived Control 103
Validity Questions 106
Summarizing the Need for Change 108
Steps to Implementation 110
Final Summary 122

Appendix of Figures

Appendix 1: Intervention Points in the Health Belief Model 127
Appendix 2: Points Where Sanitarians Can Influence
              Decision Making 129
Appendix 3: Evaluation Interviews 130
Appendix 4: Evaluation Checklist 133
Appendix 5: Sanitarian's Checklist 135

ABSTRACT

Environmental health concerns[1] are strongly linked to the occurrence of illness and contagion, events with serious implications for community public health. Why don't people correct these conditions? Persistence of noncompliance, even after the use of legal interventions, raises doubt about the efficacy of the service program and the sanitarian. This makes exploratory research for alternate explanations worthwhile.

Public health professionals usually dismiss the need for research as irrelevant or moot. There are any number of explanations for this perspective, some justified, some not. Many sanitarians view noncompliant behavior as recalcitrant and psychologically motivated; under that premise, causality is inaccessible to analysis or intervention. In any event, regardless of cause, the main task is problem resolution or abatement: causality is a moot point. "Reasonable" people comply with the law, indicating that the needed tools and resources are available. Given the proper incentive, the noncompliant will correct their behavior. Enforcement-based interventions are, therefore, the best recourse to raise fear levels and gain compliance.

Yet noncompliance continues. Short-term compliance lapses or is replaced by new cases of noncompliance. People who appear "reasonable" still cannot find a way to comply, even in the face of legal mandate. Furthermore, the use of legal enforcement and fear arousal techniques isolate sanitarians and transform them into a displeasing police presence.

These concerns indicate the need for an alternative explanation and a more efficacious intervention strategy, one including both psychological (inner-driven) and environmental (external) causal factors. Resolving even one noncompliance case is significant if it prevents illness and makes

---

[1] Imminent, critical concerns such as unsafe food temperatures in food service, inadequate water disinfection in swimming pools or contaminated drinking water are the main focus in this book. These concerns present a higher relative public health risk than infrastructural concerns (e.g. equipment repair, structural defects) and have a straight forward, behaviorally based compliance strategy (put foods in the refrigerator or on ice, add chlorine to swimming pool water and so forth).

David Mikkola, R.S., M.P.H.

services more efficacious; abatement prior to the use of enforcement releases resources for other applications, retains the client's commitment to public health and creates impetus for future compliance.

This book offers a framework for this strategy, using behavioral science concepts to offer alternative explanations of noncompliance. Then, after suggesting why people do not comply, there are ideas for changing education programs, communication campaigns and intervention strategies.

While this research is decades old, it is new to the environmental health profession. The attempt here is to adapt it to the sanitarian's needs, to suggest a framework for thinking about, and better understanding, the process of noncompliance.

The Health Belief Model and other behavioral science concepts are offered as discussion benchmarks; these tools, supplemented with public health networking, might allow sanitarians to better anticipate noncompliance motivators. Recommendations are provided for more effective site inspections, better public health networking and more consistent compliance.

FROM THE AUTHOR

I worked as an environmental health professional for thirty-one years at county health agencies. From the start, I wondered why clients did not comply with seemingly logical, commonsense regulations. Compliance seemed easy, at least with these rules; why did clients persist, even to the point of verbally attacking sanitarians and inviting the removal of their operations license? From the start, the answers given by public health professionals were all the same: clients know the rules and have the resources, but refuse to act. Legal enforcement is needed to motivate compliance. The word *recalcitrant* was the main talking point in this explanation. The predominant action was to use fear arousal and enforcement techniques. No other possible responses were explored.

This explanation seemed inadequate; it was not supported by field observations. Some clients clearly resisted change; they could reasonably be labeled 'recalcitrant'. However, in too many cases, work experience did not support the ideas that (a) noncompliant people were lazy, ignorant, or recalcitrant; (b) information and resources for compliance were readily available; and (c) given enough legal enforcement, clients would be fearful and anxious enough to change behaviors. I observed reasonable, informed clients who tried to comply, even under the duress of legal action. In some cases, they were confused; in others, they could not find the information and resources needed to comply. In contrast to these individuals, there were truly recalcitrant clients who literally laughed their way through an enforcement proceeding that, while giving some fleeting punishment, ultimately allowed them to obtain another operating license to continue their noncompliance.

Coincidental with this enforcement based view of noncompliance was a preoccupation with data collection and report generation, seemingly for its own sake. The report was the focus of the site visit, not a comprehensive evaluation of processes. The resulting list of violations, with no consideration of site trends and developments, seemed to antagonize clients even more and exacerbate the noncompliance problem.

I was not the only one affected by these concerns. New sanitarians arrived on staff, motivated to produce meaningful work, only to succumb to apathy. Attempts to find other explanations or approaches to the problem were deemed a waste of time and resources. In sum, the problem of noncompliance was not being explained or addressed effectively.

That is the reason for this book, a search for a more comprehensive explanation. During my public health academic work, I first heard of the Health Belief Model, a model that provided a more comprehensive explanation of noncompliant behavior. I was instructed by one of its authors, whose enthusiasm convinced me of its importance. There were theories such as the Social Learning Theory, McGuire's communication matrix, and Fishbein and Ajzen's Reasoned Action Approach, and considerable research on the effects of fear arousal; combined they offered ideas for expanding intervention designs beyond the use of legal enforcement.

While my supervisors at work viewed these concepts as 'ivory tower' thinking, one health educator was applying the concepts in her work. Perhaps these ideas were more than academic thinking? A few sanitarians were trying to talk with their clients, to expand their inspections beyond note taking and report generation. This convinced me that these ideas had useful applications for sanitarians.

I began searching for a better explanation and intervention design to influence environmental health decision making. Two phases of this thinking include this book and an environmental health consulting service—DJM Food Service Associates. The consulting service tries to provide a holistic comprehensive service that integrates behavioral science concepts with the existing system. The book sketches the framework for further inquiries about environmental noncompliance, a combination of health behavior concepts with the holistic concepts already taught in college to environmental health and natural science students. Along the way, I suggest how sanitarians can use these concepts in their work. Further research will be needed to proceed past this stage in thinking.

This book is based on thirty-one years of public health work in Michigan. While this experience was extensive and recent, conditions may have changed since that time. Descriptions and conclusions are based on observations from that work; some information from food codes may be different in the reader's geographical area. Limited space and resources demand some general conclusions; there will always be exceptions to any rule. Experiences, processes and applications of behavioral science may differ elsewhere.

A word of caution is important to end this section. While behavioral science theories and models are cited in the pages ahead, the purpose is not to claim a scientifically relevant application. Rather, there are three reasons for this writing: to introduce sanitarians to, what is for them, new information about learning and decision making; to suggest ways the information can be integrated into environmental heath activities; and last, to propose a framework for further discussion and research. The Health Belief Model is still being researched after sixty-odd years of work; just as much research, and more, will be needed on the ideas in this book.

So many sanitarians, with few exceptions, work hard every day to protect their communities and help clients improve their public health status. It is a difficult task. This book is an attempt to help that process. I thank the readers for listening.

Please contact the author with questions or comments: dmikkola@gmail.com. Camera-ready, *pdf* copies of forms are available at a minimal charge: contact the author.

THE INSPECTION-BASED ENFORCEMENT APPROACH TO NONCOMPLIANCE

The inspection-based enforcement system has positive, necessary aspects, aspects that will make change, however important, slow and incremental. Here is a synopsis of the process, provided for non-sanitarians and to establish a common ground for discussion[2].

The sanitarian's task is to evaluate sites and facilities for public health risk factors (the latter are established by legal mandate, varying degrees of severity and epidemiological association with environmental concerns [illness, contamination]) and take action to abate those risks. Available time and resources are oriented around documenting risk conditions and producing a complete, objective report of these findings. Data about the site is gathered using a wide range of equipment such as meters, test kits, thermometers, measuring tapes, levels and probes; computers are used to document findings and create a report. Last, site personnel are observed on the job and interviewed, to determine their knowledge, skills and abilities to apply safe sanitation procedures.

The completed site report is then discussed with the client, including aspects such as (a) the site's overall sanitation status; (b) problems and their solutions, those cited on the report and developing trends the sanitarian has observed; (c) compliance times; and (d) repercussions of continued noncompliance (e.g., more frequent site visits, hearings, fines, tickets, court actions). Other notifications may be issued, such as placards or tags, if the site's status is unacceptable.

While the sanitarian specifies the end result for each citation (e.g. a floor in good repair, clean hands, clean and sanitized equipment),

---

[2] This book primarily uses examples from food service sanitation programs; the concepts apply best to ongoing, long-term service activities such as food service, health care, swimming pool use or institutional care. The concepts apply, however, to nearly every type of environmental health noncompliance.

a *specific* comprehensive method or process (e.g. linoleum, quarry or ceramic tile, texture and type of wall paint, precise methods for washing hands or cleaning equipment) may not always be stated. Such descriptions take space on the report, take time to write and may exclude a method better suited for the client and site. Too much detail could cost the facility added expense, yield a worse result or give the client an excuse to delay compliance. This is an important point in the compliance process; clients and site personnel must be educated and experienced enough to institute changes that are legal, correct and best suited for their facility.

After the initial site evaluation, the sanitarian monitors the site's progress toward compliance, using site visits, telephone calls, correspondence and office conferences, until acceptable sanitation status is achieved. Secondary functions to the site visit include consultations, conferences, educational programs and other resources[3], to clarify report results and corresponding coping strategies. If return visits demonstrate a significant risk reduction, the sanitarian moves to another site and client. If, however, items of significant risk continue to be cited, return site visits occur, using progressively more severe legal remedies (tickets, fines, license revocation, injunctions) until these items are resolved. If necessary, action is taken to remove the offending site or facility from operation. This is an entirely different process, involving additional legal hearings, the gathering of evidence, and the writing of reports.

Considerable time, training, and resources are devoted, not only to producing an objective, comprehensive report but also to maintain and calibrate the equipment needed for the job, Note that this equipment is vital, not just to gather data, but to produce an accurate report with legal standing.

Aside from the legal mandate, and the sanitarian's essential role as environmental protector, this report is important for political, professional and legal reasons. Detached observation, along with the use of progressively more complicated equipment, gives the sanitarian

---

[3] There are two "clients" involved here, the general public using the site and site personnel serving the public. Both groups use the site services and may comingle. The term "client" implies a service-oriented, protective function not an adversarial one.

credibility as a scientist and technician. A complete and comprehensive report is a more reliable legal document. The public sees such a document as evidence that tax dollars are used constructively. The failure to produce such a report could result in legal liabilities, citations for professional malfeasance, or much worse, the loss of operating funds due to a failed audit. The time, resources, and professional pride involved in creating this "product" reflect the investment health agencies have in this system.

Note: This book makes frequent references to repeat contact with clients. It might appear, therefore, that single visit services such as water well and septic system evaluations would not apply. That is not the case, however. Repeat contacts are not just site visits but may include any contact between the client and health agency personae (printed literature, media releases, communication campaigns, school system curricula, local fairs, exhibitions or festivals, and word of mouth reports from other clients or visits to nurses, doctors, dentists, hospitals or clinics). Any of these contacts will influence the health agency's credibility as well as the client's motivation to act, perhaps even more so than direct contact with a sanitarian.

SUPPORT FOR THE INSPECTION SYSTEM

The description above illustrates the considerable pride and investment sanitarians have in what they see as objective, balanced, and scientific work. Most sanitarians working with public agencies do so to serve the community; if money rather than professional pride was the main reason for working, private industry offers sanitarians a larger income. Therefore, suggestions of bias or harassment receive a dim view, similar to a patient's questioning of a physician's regimen. The sanitarian's academic training[4] and professional orientation both advocate a balanced holistic environmental approach to problems[5]: sanitarians believe[6] that they are reflecting that ideal in their work (Fig. 1).

---

[4] See Figure 1: the *E*'s represent a holistic approach toward environmental problem solving: three factors receive different emphases depending on the situation and the client. The concept is taught in environmental health curricula, setting the sanitarian's profession apart from other natural scientists.

[5] The three *E*'s approach is still important enough to define the profession. Current hiring practices, however, emphasize a wider range of academic disciplines, resulting in an inconsistent mix of components and an inconsistent intervention strategy.

[6] While this belief is sincere and an integral part of the profession, it is distorted by sociopolitical pressures and misconceptions about human health behavior, the main tenet of this book.

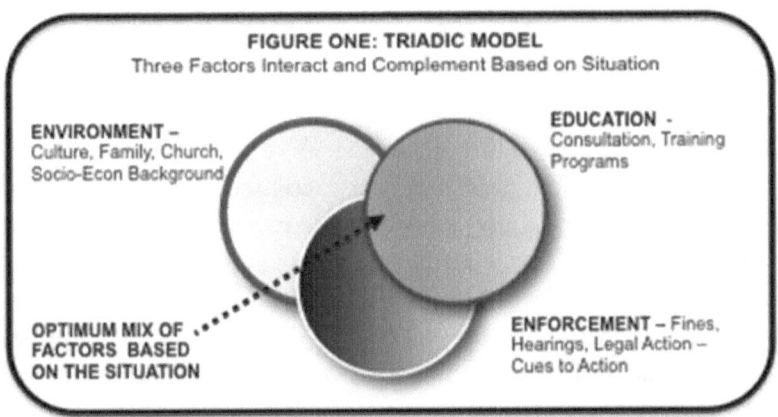

To some extent, their belief is supported: there is compelling evidence of this approach. Most public health regulations are clear, logical, well publicized, and, with the exception of more complicated upgrades to structure or equipment, easily resolved through behavioral change. There are education programs, media releases, newsletters, and pamphlets to explain the rules[7]. Many clients comply without legal pressures, indicating a good understanding of public health requirements or at least an effective use of information about them. The inspection process is the same approach used by other civil authorities (e.g., police, fire, municipal) and therefore is familiar to the community. If there are to be errors in the use of the system, it certainly appears more prudent to be too severe and be certain imminent high-risk violations are found and abated. Tentativeness caused by being familiar with clients or discussing improvements could inadvertently create confusion and encourage noncompliance.[8]

More anecdotal supportive evidence comes from field experience. Regular, repeated observations of high risk concerns lead sanitarians to believe that a client's excuses must be irrational or inexplicable, i.e. psychological in nature. This makes some sense: thinking about the

---

[7] Public health agencies believe that they are providing effective education; therefore, they believe clients cannot use ignorance as an excuse for noncompliance. This error is corrected later in this book.

[8] Supervision and audit standards give this reason for not allowing positive comments on inspection reports.

costs and potential impact of food borne illness, who can conceive of a rational explanation for statistically significant causal factors such as improper hand washing?

Yet, these repeat occurrences appear to indicate a significant disconnect between site personnel and accepted scientific knowledge. When confronted with these concerns, clients are frustrated, apologetic and mystified about their occurrence; this suggests, again, that no good explanation exists, at least not to the client and certainly not to the sanitarian. From these observations evolves the idea that either the causes are psychological and inexplicable or simply recalcitrant, i.e. not the fault of inefficacious environmental health services.

Compliance with *infrastructural* defects (e.g., floors, walls, or equipment in disrepair) is more complicated than high risk-behavioral concerns, due to strong causal links to environmental factors such as resources, time, cost or availability. The most motivated client may find barriers to change overwhelming and out of their control. High-risk *behavioral* concerns, however, while certainly linked to environmental barriers, are much less resource dependent[9]. Proper hand washing, utensil washing, and food storage are three commonly accepted hygienic practices, at home or in restaurants. From the sanitarian's perspective, the *rational* approach to this type of violation should be staff training and routine monitoring of the problem. Since this does not require a significant investment of resources, at least from the sanitarian's perspective, training should happen and compliance should occur. On that basis, noncompliance must be *irrational* and recalcitrant[10] behavior. (This book will try to suggest a different approach).

---

[9] While it could be argued that infrastructure influences behavior (a hand sink must be convenient and operational for hand washing to occur; a building must be in good repair to allow efficient operations), individual volition and behavior (proper and frequent use of the sink) remain the primary driving forces.

[10] *Recalcitrant* def.—"having an obstinately uncooperative attitude toward authority or discipline." (Apple computer software dictionary); "resisting authority, hard to . . . handle" (Microsoft Word dictionary). The temptation to categorize all noncompliance in this manner leads to overreliance on the use of enforcement.

Furthermore, the sanitarian's *primary* function, defined and driven by legal mandate, is always risk abatement, not analysis. This function is locked in by legal mandate and community demand. Documentation and corrective action remain the foundation of the legal mandate and matching funds requirements, not the analysis of noncompliance. If a sanitarian is intent on learning a client's motivations, more time must be generated during the site visit, not an easy proposition.[11] While some sanitarians persist in this effort, administrators generally discourage this effort as moot, a waste of time and resources. Since causes of noncompliance must be irrational and recalcitrant (at least under the present system), analysis is futile. Analysis does not contribute anything toward risk abatement[12]. To its advocates, the inspection system has worked well to limit the impact of overt public health problems[13]; any noncompliance not covered by existing enforcement can be accredited either to the client's recalcitrance or the need for more stringent inspections[14].

The inspection-based system and its corresponding view of noncompliant behavior as recalcitrant are both supported by public health administrators, the public, the sanitarian's anecdotal field experience, and the literature; thus sanitarians are reluctant to change the system. In addition, external audits and associated budget dollars are linked to the system.

Even if these audits did *not* exist, however, public health professionals would still be comfortable with the system. The public and many clients see the system as an efficient use of tax dollars and a fair, equitable

---

[11] Ideas on how to do this will come later.

[12] It does, however, yield important information about long term compliance and intervention design

[13] Imminent concerns such as epidemics or contagion. These concerns are *not* the subject of this book: they are adequately addressed through the use of enforcement. At issue here are environmental health concerns that are predominantly chronic and subclinical, developing over some time. The latter are not recognized or addressed in endemic mode; the system does not have the tools to do so.

[14] Administrators respond to persistent noncompliance by *increasing* legal penalties and enforcement accessories (e.g. tickets, fines, having sanitarians wear uniforms or carry badges)

administration of the law. Historically, sanitarians have been expected to contain the spread of imminent public health hazards (e.g., tuberculosis, community disasters), as in the case of epidemics or communitywide contamination.

The public expects this protective function and looks for legal actions as an effective use of tax dollars. A comprehensive site report of sanitary violations feeds into this expectation. Anecdotal field experience shows the citation of severe sanitation risks, providing enough evidence to support this system. Finally, the system provides respect for the sanitarian's professional development as a scientist and technician. Each site report supplies a viable legal document and establishes credibility and respect for the sanitarian. (Professional respect is vital when competing for a portion of a shrinking public health budget.)

Public health professionals rarely cite literature to support their system; this may explain why assumptions about noncompliance are based on field experience,[15] not on behavioral science. Conceptual explanations, however, resemble psychodynamic[16] theory. This theory states that noncompliant or "deviant" behavior is attributed to a "manifestation of the dynamic interplay of inner forces, most of which operate below the level of consciousness."[17] "Causes of noncompliance are thought to be psychological, hidden and unavailable for further inquiry. The sanitarian's perspective is based on outcome, not cause (the cause in this case, by definition, is within the individual, unavailable for inquiry). This fact forces further use of legal enforcement to influence outcome.

---

[15] The lack of exploratory research is often used as an excuse for not changing the system.

[16] While this theory may never have officially been cited by health professionals, it closely resembles the rationale and explanation given for noncompliant behavior. While there are exceptions to every rule, the author has never heard a public health administrator acknowledge the role of environmental causal factors in noncompliant behavior. It was rare, in the author's career at least, to see public health literature or education programs present concerns in a persuasive tone.

[17] Albert Bandura, *Social Foundations of Thought & Action: A Social Cognitive Theory* (Englewood Cliffs, New Jersey: Prentice-Hall, Inc. 1986) p. 2

A CRITIQUE OF THE SYSTEM

The preceding section describes necessary parts of the inspection- and enforcement-based system, why it seems perfectly justified, and how it has become entrenched in the public health psyche. This lengthy discussion was needed to illustrate the deep investment sanitarians have in the system and the difficulty of subsequent change, however warranted. As with any attempt at change, there will be individuals reluctant to endorse it. In line with behavioral science concepts, potential objections to change must be addressed. After that, we can examine why these changes are important and necessary.

CONSIDERING OBJECTIONS TO CHANGE

As a precursor to a critique of the system, we need to consider why public health professionals might not endorse a systemic change (later, there will be specific changes to consider). There are several possible reasons: (a) there is no research to suggest there is a problem; (b) if there were problems, solutions must originate with legislators, not sanitarians; and (c) there has not been prior criticism of the system.

It is true that there is no exploratory research; this is unlikely to change until a crisis highlights problems with the system. The emphasis of current environmental health service is *retroactive*, not proactive. This is due to legislative mandate, budget constraints, sociopolitical pressures and the nature of the science itself. Administrators are reluctant to budget exploratory research that is expensive to conduct and difficult to justify. Environmental concerns are subclinical or chronic, not acute as with the work of doctors or nurses. Any documentation is often biased, relying on a self-interested client's report or on anecdotal evidence. Since problems are difficult to document, the not entirely unreasonable assumption is that they do not exist.

Legislative mandates restrict the sanitarian's options during inspections, locking in certain enforcement-based components to the inspection and written report (see "The Inspection-Based Enforcement Approach"). While program funding is linked to satisfying these mandates, however, these restrictions should not be an excuse to avoid changes to the system or to resist screening for developing trends. A certain amount of reluctance is understandable; however, there still is ample room within the existing system to incorporate the changes suggested in this book. Once these improvements are instituted and documented by research, public pressure may cause legislators to amend the system.

While there is little concrete data to use in program evaluation, there is compelling anecdotal information and personal experience to suggest the need for change. Many individuals have experiences in which they act contrary to legal mandates, friends' advice, or scientific research. Other factors or information influence their decision. Similarly, sanitarians see clients who, faced with legal action, still are unable to rectify violations: these people appear reasonable and sincere yet cannot make the required changes. They simply do not fit the expected "recalcitrant" stereotype.

Finally, critics use the absence of supporting data or research to suggest that these ideas are overemphasized and unrealistic, and are the work of "ivory tower" academics. However, if this discussion is new to sanitarians, it is *not* new to health educators or behavioral scientists. In 1975, Goldsmith and Hochbaum observed the shortcomings of environmental protection, stating that

> Neither strict enforcement of environmental codes nor concerted consumer education has prevent people from subjecting the environment to continuous insults, even though these insults will be to their ultimate detriment. Yet these measures have been the main ones on which public health environmentalists have relied in their environmental protection efforts.

The authors suggest a reason why these 'insults' continue and why sanitarians do not change their approach: "they (sanitarians) have been trained to deal primarily with the symptoms or the results . . . rather than with the determinants of human behavior."[18] They go on to decry the lack of available information for motivated clients wishing to comply, stating that "environmental health agencies . . . have all too often made information available only to those who know where to obtain it and are willing to make the effort to do so."[19] This would suggest that some changes and exploratory research are needed to explore both behavioral science applications and the nature of consumer education.

---

[18] Francis J. Goldsmith, Godfrey M. Hochbaum, "Changing People's Behavior Toward the Environment," *Public Health Reports*, May-June 1975, 90(3): quote on p. 231 article pp. 231-234.

[19] Francis J. Goldsmith, Godfrey M. Hochbaum, "Changing People's Behavior Toward the Environment," *Public Health Reports*, May-June 1975, 90(3): pp,.231-234 quote p. 232

THE PROFESSION'S DEVELOPMENT AND MINDSET

Sanitarians might not want to consider changes to what seems to be an age-old, established system. While the system appears mandated, without possibility of change, it is foreign to the sanitarian's academic and historical professional development. Examination of this original intellectual foundation indicates that a more general, holistic system might be more professionally comfortable and change might not be as difficult or traumatic as imagined.

For, while the sanitarian's essential role appears to be that of enforcement officer, in actuality, their professional and intellectual evolution closely parallels the behavioral science theories presented in this book. While it could be argued that these theories are idealistic, unattainable thinking, they reflects the thinking of today's sanitarian, *absent the constraints of socio-political barriers to change*. Most sanitarians believe, for example, that they practice a holistic, triadic approach toward resolving noncompliance. They shun the idea of being an enforcement officer and promote communication and education as their chief 'enforcement' tools. Moving toward the latter functions may not only be more effective but also a more pleasing and comfortable role to assume.

A key definition of environmental health, advanced by the World Health Organization, reflects this idea, that enforcement is only one of ten major factors in the profession (Figure 2)

> Environmental health addresses all the physical, chemical, and biological factors external to a person, and all the related factors impacting behaviors. It encompasses the assessment and control of those environmental factors that can potentially affect health. It is targeted toward preventing disease and creating health-supportive environments.[20]

---

20   http://www.who.int/topics/environmental_health/en/—While the definition excludes some types of health behaviors, it includes words such as *control* and *potentially*; i.e. a holistic approach to the profession.

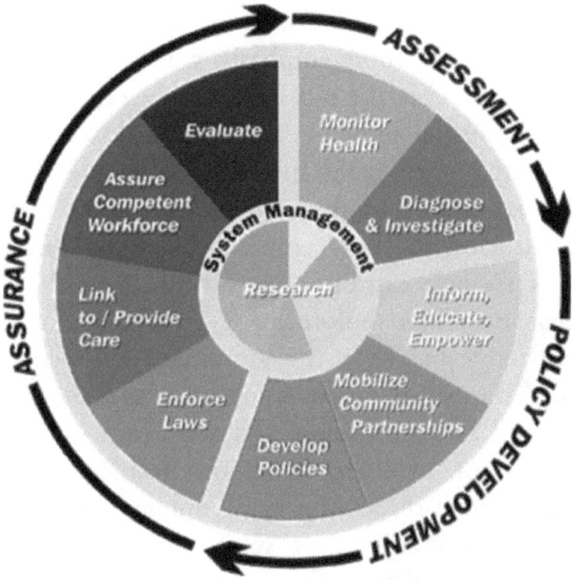

Figure 2: American Public Health Association's "Ten Essential Public Health Services". Enforcement is only one. [Footnote 10]

In this way, sanitarians *guard* the environmental community, using enforcement sparingly and only when required. Figure 2 also shows this holistic perspective; enforcement is one of ten public health functions, a reasonable and restrained[21] approach. All avenues of persuasion are explored.[22]

This definition underscores not only the importance of "abatement" but also proactive "assessment" and "prevention" of illness and contagion. In turn, the objective in figure 1 is, rather than to rely on enforcement techniques alone, to create an optimum mix of factors, situation specific, such that the client is *persuaded* to change behaviors. Thus, depending

---

[21] See the American Public Health Association's website, http://www.apha.org/programs/standards/, for the text; graphic is produced on Community Tool Box website, http://ctb.ku.edu/ Sanitarians believe in an approach based on field experience and prevailing attitudes, perpetuated by task delineation and bureaucratic structuring. Research of social psychologists and behavioral scientists relate different conclusions; *that* research is the foundation of this book.

[22] This is the key phrase; this book suggests that, while all tools are used, they are not used to their fullest extent.

on the client's mind set and the facility situation, one of the three factors might receive more emphasis, while implying use of the other two. On the return visit, the mix might change completely.

American public health historical development reflects this holism, an attempt to avoid specialists who might emphasize one perspective or explanation at the expense of another. Hardly a recent discussion, Shattuck, an early American public health pioneer, argued for professionals capable of resolving any sort of health concern. Within that paradigm, enforcement is balanced with the need to persuade and educate. Thus the sanitarian developed historically as a *mix* of professions: an epidemiologist *as well as* an enforcer, an investigator as well as an evaluator and scientist[23]. While enforcement was clearly important to abate sanitation problems in an expanding industrial base, the early architects of public health argued for considering all explanations and causes. While there are many historical examples of this thinking, two more famous ones are the London cholera outbreak and

---

[23] Historically, the sanitarian's profession is defined as a compromise between the physician and the police officer. See the following: (1) Lemuel Shattuck, *Report of the Sanitary Commission of the State of Massachusetts—1850* (http://www.deltaomega.org/documents/shattuck.pdf) warns against the sanitarian as "specialist," arguing that ". . . the Board should be able to bring competent knowledge to the investigation of every subject . . . [and] the idea . . . that everything relating to health belongs exclusively to one profession, operates against sanitary improvement. The services of medical men are indispensable; but the services of other professions, and of every person in their respective spheres must be put in requisition, before reform can be complete" (p. 75). Shattuck then goes on to describe the composition of the Board of Health. Regarding the role of enforcement, he argues, consistent with the argument in this book, that ". . . we recommend that local Boards of Health endeavor to carry into effect all their orders and regulations in a conciliatory manner; and that they resort to compulsory process only when the public good requires it" (p. 81)

Typhoid Mary.[24] [25] While enforcement played a vital role in abatement (e.g. removing Mary from food service, removing the London water well pump handle), it took skilled investigators to initially determine and find the contamination sources.

Academia also reflects this holistic perspective. Environmental health curricula instruct sanitarians, rather than work *retrospectively* from known risk factors to infer and expect problems (and statistically established solutions), to evaluate situations as they exist and formulate solutions based on a spectrum of observed causes and concerns. All stakeholders and interests are represented, and the intervention is comprehensive and innovative. Problems are explored that might not have been analyzed using a narrow list of established risk factors. (This perspective, again, is reflected in figure 1).

In contrast, the existing system emphasizes retrospective, after-the-fact assessment of the presence of abstract risk factors. The main emphasis is abatement of *outcome* behavior, not evaluation of that behavior's evolution or underlying causality. Since sanitarians come to a site armed with expected causes and risk factors, there are unexplained cases of noncompliance evolving, endemic or even epidemic contagions left undetected. The site report is generated based on preset risk factors, not the evaluation of systems and processes.

While the existing system is effective for abating short-term[26] overt public health concerns, other concerns continue overtly but also in an endemic or subclinical fashion. Critical, high-risk hazards such as poor personal hygiene continue and even increase.[27] In that instance, the

---

[24] Judith Walzer Leavitt, "Typhoid Mary: Villain or Victim?" http://www.pbs.org/wgbh/nova/body/typhoid-mary-villain-or-victim.html

[25] UCLA Department of Epidemiology, "Who is John Snow?" http://www.ph.ucla.edu/epi/snow.html

[26] The sanitarian's work appears "short-term" due to artificial work divisions (brief geographical assignments, limited time for site inspections) for accounting purposes. The client perceives these services much differently, however.

[27] While statistics fluctuate over time, by one estimate, one-third of foodborne illness cases are attributed to poor personal hygiene (www.cdc.gov) In the time period of 1990-97, viral foodborne cases rose by ten times

convenient location and proper outfitting of hand wash sinks ignores the importance of behavioral science in assuring their consistent use. Long-term habits do not change; a comprehensive explanation would address *both* short- and long-term impacts.

Psychologists criticize the inspection system's underlying scientific assumption, psychodynamic theory, on the grounds that it is both an incomplete and a retrospective explanation of noncompliant behavior. Faced with a decision to act, and in the presence of a constant psychological influence (e.g., legal threats and fear arousal), people motivated to act properly may pay more attention to, and be influenced by *environmental* factors (opinions of significant others, resources and skills needed to act, perceived barriers or obstacles to action). The presence of the psychological causal factor *may or may not* predict the final behavior; other motivators must be included in an intervention paradigm. While emotion heightens awareness of the need to act, that internal factor does not motivate consistently enough to be the foundation of an intervention. Fear and anxiety work on people in different ways. According to Bandura,

> An internal motivator cannot adequately account for marked shifts in a given behavior under differing situational circumstances. When varying social conditions produce predictable changes in behavior, the postulated cause cannot reside mainly in a drive in the organism . . . (further) behavior patterns commonly attributed to unconscious inner causes can be instated, eliminated and reinstated by varying appropriate social influences . . . . [28]

---

while bacterial cases decreased fourfold. (US Centers for Disease Control, *Morbidity and Mortality Weekly Report*, 6/12/09, 58(22 609-615).

[28] Psychological explanations of noncompliance are incomplete without consideration of environmental influences. Albert Bandura, *Social Foundations of Thought & Action: A Social Cognitive Theory* (Englewood Cliffs, New Jersey: Prentice-Hall, 1986), quote from pp. 2-3, further discussion on pp. 2-4 (a critique of psychodynamic theory and psychological motivators). Also see Albert Bandura, *Social Learning*

Thus people gain weight, continue smoking, disregard traffic rules, or fail to wash soiled hands in the face of various levels of fear. Or perhaps they change behaviors due to *environmental* causes or information from those sources, *independent* of any *psychological* causes. So, when a client attributes noncompliance to factors external to his or her control, this complaint may be more than just an excuse: it might be worthy of consideration.

Sanitarians see noncompliant clients who cannot comply, to the point of losing their operating license or going to jail. That certainly is inexplicable behavior in and of itself; some other cause must be driving those decisions. If environmental influences can influence and produce noncompliant behavior commonly attributed to inner-based causes, why limit the design of intervention? That being said, we continue on to consider the other areas where the system is lacking.

Another objection to the psychodynamic, recalcitrant perspective is that it does not fit well with the sanitarian's image as public health teacher and guardian. Most sanitarians do not feel comfortable with an enforcement-based persona; they see this police image as incompatible with the public health mission.[29] Theories and interventions advanced in support of the profession should not create cognitive dissonance or professional discomfort for sanitarians. The image of a sanitarian on every street corner holding a shield and wearing a uniform should give pause: if this is required to gain lasting compliance, is it worthwhile? Perhaps it is needed for a public health emergency, but is it desirable on a long-term basis? There must be other options to gain compliance.

Theory (Englewood Cliffs, New Jersey: Prentice-Hall, 1977) for a general discussion—Ch. 1 pp. 2-13

[29] See figure 2 above and the linked website.

William James reflects this idea when he states that

> when we make theories about the world . . . we do so in order to attain a conception . . . which shall give us subjective satisfaction. And, if there be two conceptions, and the one seems to us . . . more rational than the other, we are entitled to suppose that the more rational one is truer of the two.[30]

While philosophers dismiss this argument as whimsy (and public health administrators may dismiss it as whining), there is logic to it; between two nearly identical arguments, it makes sense to choose the one that is a better fit with our experience, with which we feel more comfortable and compatible. While choosing the negative, unpleasant persona posed by enforcement might be effective in the midst of environmental contamination or an illness outbreak, it is definitely not the image people envision from a public health agency. Neither is it the image most sanitarians would choose. The subjectively satisfying feeling cannot help but impact the sanitarian's morale and motivation.

Decades of behavioral science research prove a strong link between perception of reality and actual behavior for individuals contemplating behavioral change. Similarly, the efficacy of any intervention will be influenced by the morale and perceptions of those administering it. The excessive or inappropriate use of fear arousal can be both detrimental to long-term compliance strategies and aesthetically displeasing and demoralizing for those administering the intervention. No matter the potential effectiveness of an intervention design, an uncomfortable or demoralized professional may inadvertently cause the intervention to fail.

At some point in every intervention, noncompliant behavior is resolved, if only to remove the client from operation. The question is the associated cost in letting the legal intervention continue on so long, especially if there are other tools that might shorten the process. What

---

[30] William James, "The Dilemma of Determinism," in *A Modern Introduction to Philosophy*, 3rd ed., Edwards and Papp, editors (New York: The Free Press, 1973), p. 35.

is the cost in morale, public relations, psychology, public health, and politics?

The major concerns with the existing system are (a) an overemphasis on the use of legal enforcement as the *only* intervention; (b) the failure to proactively communicate and educate; and (c) the sanitarian's progressively negative enforcement image.

The premise of this book is that accepted explanations of noncompliant behavior and associated interventions have been ineffective in producing *lasting* change in a statistically significant number of cases. While short-term compliance inevitably occurs as a result of fear arousal and legal enforcement, and while the public appears to appreciate this perceived progress, it is not without costs (economic, public relations, political, professional). As compliance created through the use of fear arousal decays, discouraged and embittered clients may relapse into previous noncompliant behaviors or even engage in new violations unaddressed by the site report. Since the emphasis on enforcement efforts has diverted resources and skills away from education and consultation functions, the latter are only marginally effective when called upon for use. Finally, the sanitarian's persona as legal enforcer is inappropriate and displeasing within service-oriented public health venues. It positions public health as an enforcement- and adversarial-based profession, not as a positive service for reducing public health risk.

OVER EMPHASIS ON LEGAL ENFORCEMENT

A major objection to the inspection system, voiced by the public and sanitarians alike, is the *over*emphasis on the use of legal enforcement. To some extent, legally mandated rules lock sanitarians into this mode. External audits, and associated matching fund awards, require that (a) public health risk[31] has been evaluated accurately and completely; (b) the sanitarian has interviewed site personnel and evaluated their skills and knowledge; and (c) a report has been issued in the proper format, detailing sanitation concerns and the legal repercussions of continued noncompliance.[32]

At this point, however, these rules all too often produce unwanted, negative effects. Attention to comprehensive reporting and documentation, while essential for legal purposes, also has side effects of escalating the client's fear and tension, as well as taking precious resources away from holistic analysis of the site's sanitation status.

Clients begin to orient themselves to the presence or absence of legal enforcement rather than the existing sanitation concerns[33]. The site report and associated punitive actions drive the client's motivation to act and perceptions both of their self-efficacy and the facility's sanitation status. In some cases, punitive actions and the client's reactions may accelerate the effect, to the extent that 'elevated levels of anxiety . . . far exceed the fear experienced during the actual threatening situation'[34]. A more comprehensive, multi-faceted intervention might have diluted this effect.

---

[31] Checklist items have varying degrees of risk but are statistically related to disease etiology by the Centers for Disease Control and Prevention.

[32] This is a summary of the main concerns, taken from the author's memory as a sanitarian.

[33] During a food service consultation, the author noted a sanitation concern and included it on his report to the client. The client dismissed this stating that since the health department sanitarian had not cited it, it was not a problem.

[34] Albert Bandura, "Self-efficacy: Toward a Unifying Theory of Behavioral Change" *Psychological Review* V. 84 (7) 1977 pp. 191-215 quote on p. 199

The evaluation and associated report must be complete and correct, leaving less time for the client's questions and concerns[35]. The process of writing, editing and printing a report, not the overall site status, becomes the focus of the site visit for the sanitarian and site personnel. Interviews focus on collecting information about unobserved or potential violations, not discussions of improvements or positive developments. Site personnel may seem defensive, anxious and guilty, as they work to explain problems they may not have observed[36].

Within this context, sanitarians are easily predisposed to see unsanitary conditions, even if only partially developed (auditors are critical when a concern is missed), and to be negatively biased in site and personnel assessments. Audit demands, coupled with time and resource constraints, produce a restricted microcosm based on an artificial checklist of sanitation concerns. For example, the report must include the legal repercussions of further noncompliance but only recommends reinforcing positive sanitation trends. Since future visits are built upon this initial benchmark, subsequent evaluations reference only the presence or absence of *previously* cited risk factors.[37] Noncompliance becomes a self-fulfilling prophecy, with each visit documenting risk relative to the initial evaluation. As a further consequence, the sanitarian's role is further restricted to that of enforcement officer.

As a further consequence of relying on only one intervention tool, improvements in sanitation status, presumably based on anxiety, may quickly relapse after fears have subsided. Clients learn to adjust their compliance efforts to the sanitarian's schedule. As one client told the author, as they observed a violation, 'That wasn't a violation last week when you *should* have been here! You're late!' This "roller-coaster", compliance-lapse fluctuation is due to having only one tool for intervention.

---

[35] It is ironic that when sites have greater sanitation concerns, progressively more time is needed to state this fact on a report: less time is available to discuss problem resolution.

[36] The violation may have occurred elsewhere in the facility or be based on employee interviews about prospective, unobserved behaviors. If management accompanies the sanitarian, each concern can be addressed as it is observed.

[37] A sanitarian's proactive attempt to evaluate other aspects, negative and positive, may even be challenged as an extension of his or her authority.

Legal mandates and limited resources force sanitarians to concentrate on an accurate site report, a report linked to statistically significant, established risk factors. Searching for these isolated risk factors rather than evaluating the entire site's system and processes precludes discovery of endemic or emerging sanitation trends. For example, critical violations such as improper hand washing or unsafe food temperatures may be indicators of even deeper causal concerns, i.e. inaccessible hand sinks, ineffective employee training, not enough hot or cold food storage units. Soiled utensils, a critical violation, may mask a more pervasive concern. The sanitarian should take time to delve deeper, looking at cleaning and sanitizing processes. This takes valuable time away from report generation, however.

While these criticisms should suggest the need for system reform, the system is important to public health beyond the matching budget funds provided by external audits. While strict audits are vital to assure consistent and comprehensive site reports, quantifiable results[38] (reports, correspondence, legal action) are easier to measure, have legal bearing, and appear to indicate progress. The public appreciates what is perceived to be effective use of tax monies and measurable, equitable legal administration. The system provides a comfortable professional posture for sanitarians; the emphasis on documentation and evaluation establishes them as scientists and technical advisors, giving them prestige and credibility in a competitive public health profession. So, while modifications are needed, they can occur only gradually and incrementally.

---

[38] Standards applied by Michigan State agencies are used here; since State laws are usually based on acceptance of federal codes, differences should be minimal.

EFFECTS OF FEAR AROUSAL AND ANXIETY

The emphasis on the use of enforcement creates a more significant problem: client fear arousal. While some level of fear and anxiety is unavoidable, and may even be desirable with some clients, it also can be debilitating and delay compliance in others. (This is especially true if 'the situation does not provide such alternative means to resolve . . . conflicts. . . . the person might attempt to remove himself psychologically from the conflict situation . . . (or) might be rendered incapable of thinking objectively and behaving rationally . . .'[39]). These unresolved conflicts might result in slower compliance, none at all or worse, increased **non**compliance.

Fear arousal will be present during *any* contact with sanitarians, regardless of the sanitarian's tact, the purpose of the encounter or the client's preparation, demeanor, education, or experience. This 'contact' may be real or anticipated, such as when the sanitarian is mentioned in the media or by another client, or a site evaluation is due. Even a client who is prepared for a site evaluation may still be anxious about new information or legal changes the sanitarian may discuss. While some clients probably *should* be anxious, sanitarians still need training and experience to assure effective use of fear arousal and legal protocols (warrants, injunctions).

During a site evaluation, the client receives numerous messages about their facility, messages possibly inconsistent with their knowledge and attitudes. There may be new procedures, changes in the law or previously unobserved sanitation problems in their facility. The result, *cognitive dissonance,* increases until the anxiety is resolved by accepting, rejecting or distorting the information.[40] The pressure to reduce the

---

[39] Irwin M. Rosenstock "Historical Origins of the Health Belief Model" in Marshall H. Becker, Ph.D., M.P.H. editor, *The Health Belief Model and Personal Health Behaviors* (Thorofare, New Jersey: Charles B. Slack, Inc. 1974) p. 5

[40] Dorwin Cartwright, "Some Principles of Mass Persuasion", *Human Relations*, (2), 1949, pp. 253-267.

dissonance is a "function of the magnitude of the dissonance"[41] (i.e., the credibility of the message). The sanitarian's message, if persuasive and credible[42], will produce anxiety in the client; this dissonance can be eased or avoided if "neutralizing cognitions" are available. Examples of these neutralizing ideas might be deflecting responsibility to subordinates ('good help is so hard to find'); excusing noncompliant behavior as the only choice ('everyone in the industry does the same thing', 'we don't have time or can't afford to make that change'); denying the problem's severity ('no one got sick', 'we've been doing the same thing for years') or its credibility ('that sanitarian is new or doesn't know what he's talking about', 'no one else has mentioned that problem before').[43]

> These and similar mental gymnastics enable (the client) to justify his choice between the two conflicting values, diminish his discomfort over violating one of them, and construct, so to speak, a new logical basis that fully supports his initially dubious behavioral choice. This process of rationalization leads ... to undesirable behavior (and) ... to a weakening or even to the destruction of an originally strongly held value ... we need to seek ways of preventing such a conflict initially or of effecting a different outcome. [44]

The literature is not clear as to how fear and anxiety develop and their relative impact on various clientele. For sanitarians, this point

---

[41] Martin Fishbein and Icek Ajzen *Belief, Attitude, Intention and Behavior: An Introduction to Theory and Research* (Massachusetts: Addison-Wesley, 1975), quote on p. 40, discussion of cognitive dissonance pp. 39-45.

[42] The sanitarian's training and experience, as well as the administrator's support, are critical here. Site personnel might reduce anxiety and dissonance by attempting to discrediting the message or messenger.

[43] Richard E. Petty and John T. Cacioppo. *Attitudes and Persuasion: Classic and Contemporary Approaches* (Dubuque, Iowa: Wm. C. Brown, 1981), quote from p. 145-6, entire discussion, pp. 137-152.

[44] Francis J. Goldsmith, Godfrey M. Hochbaum, "Changing People's Behavior Toward the Environment," *Public Health Reports*, May-June 1975, 90(3): pp,.231-234 quote p. 233

is as important as knowledge of the process. Some behavioral models suggest anxiety occurs in direct response to the conflicting event; others suggest the reaction could occur merely through *anticipating* the event.[45] Furthermore, the correlation, if any, to changes in behavior is unclear. To the sanitarian, the important point should be not *how* these emotions develop, *but that they exist at all. In the event that compliance is delayed or not forthcoming from a previously agreeable client, the sanitarian can look to this factor as a possible explanation.*

Every individual deals with dissonant emotions differently, depending on his or her experience, education, and attitude about the problem. As anxiety levels change, the individual acts to reduce them by changing behaviors, altering their information and attitudes about the problem, or, if they feel no viable solution is present, doing nothing. High levels of both competency and perceived self-efficacy[46] will be vital in producing the outcome important to public health. If no viable solution is at hand (i.e., the client does not see how they can cope), nothing will be done.

---

[45] http://en.wikipedia.org/wiki/Fear_appeals#The_Extended_Parallel_Process_Model. Discussion of the different fear drive models and the process of fear arousal. For more on cognitive dissonance, see Richard E. Petty and John T. Cacioppo, *Communication and Persuasion: Central and Peripheral Routes to Attitude Change* (New York: Springer-Verlag, 1986), pp. 62-63; Martin Fishbein and Icek Ajzen *Belief, Attitude, Intention and Behavior: An Introduction to Theory and Research* (Massachusetts: Addison-Wesley, 1975), pp. 39-45; Icek Ajzen and Martin Fishbein, *Understanding Attitudes and Predicting Social Behavior* (Englewood Cliffs, New Jersey: Prentice-Hall, Inc., 1980), pp. 22-23.

[46] *Self-efficacy* is defined as "the conviction that one can successfully execute the behavior required to produce the outcomes" as opposed to an outcome expectancy that "a given behavior will lead to certain outcomes" (i.e., it is viable; will relieve anxiety and fear). See Albert Bandura, *Social Learning Theory* (New Jersey: Prentice-Hall, 1977), p. 79. Discussion pp. 78-85 Self-efficacy is similar to perceived behavioral control: "I have the necessary skills and abilities to perform this behavior." Martin Fishbein and Icek Ajzen, *Predicting and Changing Behavior: The Reasoned Action Approach* (New York: Psychology Press, 2010), p. 64.

Sanitarians may be tempted, especially during stress and tense moments, to use high-fear messages to scare resistant clients into activity.[47] This may be for any number of reasons, ranging from attempts to assert authority to simply gaining the individual's attention to the message of the site visit. While "it appears that strong fear appeals and high-efficacy messages produce the greatest behavior change,"[48] to be effective and avoid an undesirable outcome, high-fear messages must be accompanied by the reassurance of coping mechanisms.[49] An individual with limited skills, education, or experience might choose to wait, hoping the "problem" will go away (i.e., the sanitarian was incorrect, a new sanitarian might ignore the violation, or needed legal enforcement might not occur) and believing there is nothing they can do to resolve the issue anyway. In contrast, someone with more experience and knowledge might attempt to discredit the message or the messenger.

These types of emotions will remain throughout the inspection and may increase as legal implications of noncompliance are discussed (as required by the audit standards), violations accumulate through the inspection, and legal citations are included with the violations on the written report. If the client is unable to reduce tension and anxiety, perhaps through the sanitarian's positive comments, negotiated extensions of compliance times or an opportunity to demonstrate facility improvements, noncompliant behavior will certainly remain and may increase as a result. Over a long time period, residual effects of any improvements will decay and resistance to further progress will build. The end result will be either a frightened client who believes compliance to be futile or impossible, or the

---

[47] Consider the sanitarian who casually opened his briefcase during a client interview, to reveal a "closed for business" placard inside. Compliance, at least for the short term, was immediate.

[48] K. Witte and M. Allen, "A Meta-Analysis of Fear Appeals: Implications for Effective Public Health Campaigns,". *Health Education & Behavior* 27(5): 591-615. Information from the abstract printed in Sage Journals website http://heb.sagepub.com/content/27/5/591. Also see Albert Bandura, *Social Learning Theory* (Englewood Cliffs, New Jersey: Prentice-Hall, 1977) p. 79.

[49] John P. Kirscht, Ph.D. "Research Related to the Modification of Health Beliefs" in Marshall H. Becker, Ph.D., M.P.H. editor, *The Health Belief Model and Personal Health Behaviors* (Thorofare, New Jersey: Charles B. Slack, Inc. 1974) p. 134

evolution of a highly resistance client previously amenable to education and consultation.

While truly recalcitrant individuals may need a strong message to prompt them to consider change, others who intend to comply may be pushed into relapse by the same message. Again, see Bandura for the failure of verbal persuasion alone:

> Efficacy expectations induced in this manner[50] are likely to be weak and short-lived. In the face of distressing threats and a long history of failure in coping with them, whatever success expectations are induced by suggestion will be rapidly extinguished by disconfirming experiences. Results of several lines of research attest to the weakness of verbal persuasion that creates expectations *without providing an authentic experiential base* . . . [51] (emphasis mine)

While a client who resists verbal persuasion may be truly recalcitrant, the explanation for failure may lie in the technique itself. The addition of a coping strategy, combined with modeling and practice, might allow the client to experience a degree of competence in handling the situation. Further, pointing out incremental improvements ("see, this part of the process is handled well; you've just got to work more on this portion" OR "let's work on this concern and I'll check back in a week; the other violations aren't as critical and they can wait") validates the client and gives him or her a reason to continue working.

In addition to the client's fears and concerns, the *sanitarian* experiences anxiety due to potential performance audits by supervisors or conflicts with the client over noncompliance. Ernest Julian suggested, at a 1984 national food conference presentation, that fewer violations may be recorded due to the attempt to avoid "confrontation between the sanitarian and operator." [52] Under this stress, sanitarians might fail to take needed legal

---

[50] i.e. verbal persuasion
[51] Albert Bandura, *Social Learning Theory* (Englewood Cliffs, New Jersey: Prentice-Hall, 1977) p. 82.
[52] Ernest M. Julian, RS, "Certification Programs: Their Effectiveness and Future: A Discussion Paper Prepared for the Second National Conference

action, sending the client a clear message that waiting may be appropriate. A consistent, credible, and community wide service program may be enough to prompt a client's attention, prior to the sanitarian's application of further fear arousal techniques.

The research is inconclusive about the effects of fear arousal in different situations and when it should be used to greatest effect. If *laboratory* research yields mixed results, the stressful site inspection environment will be even more uncertain. Therefore, to avoid the misuse of fear arousal during site visits, here are a few summary statements about its effects:

Fear arousal increases acceptance of information and the intention to act.

This is the main positive effect of fear arousal: increased attention to information, correlated attitude change, and heightened intention to act in some undetermined[53] way. Pressure brought upon the client, usually with discussion of legal consequences, increases stress and subsequent attention to the message.

Attending to information through a *strong* fear message does not necessarily prompt people to *accept, understand, learn, or retain* the information better. Janis and Feshbach state that three varying levels of fear arousal are ". . . equally effective in teaching the factual material".[54] Research suggests that

> High fear appeals . . . are effective when a readily available action can be taken to eliminate the threat, when receivers have a low anxiety personality or do not perceive themselves

---

for Food Protection," unpublished discussion paper, 1984.

[53] Raising a client's fear and anxiety may motivate them to reduce those levels; *what* they do and *how* they do it is another process, not always predictable or consistent.

[54] Irving L. Janis and Seymour Feshbach, "Effects of Fear-Arousing Communications," *Journal of Abnormal and Social Psychology*, 1953, 48(3): 78-92, 325.

as vulnerable and when a highly credible source delivers the message[55]

Most sanitarians will agree that such individuals are rare, at least in environmental health venues. In many more cases, the result of a high fear message is that "defensive avoidance may occur (thereby reducing attitude change) . . .".[56] This only serves to delay compliance and possibly damage relations between the sanitarian and site personnel. Medium or low fear arousal will be more effective; i.e., reminding clients of the *possibility* of enforcement but leaving that trump card in reserve. This approach should still produce attention to the message.[57]

The literature relates the following influential events: (1) a person's behavior is determined by their intention to perform the behavior[58]; (2) fear appeals produce more favorable attitudes[59]; and (3) "increases in fear . . . are consistently associated with increases in acceptance (intentions and behavior)".[60] Thus, a low to moderate fear appeal should ideally produce a positive change in knowledge, attitude and intention to change behaviors.

---

[55] Charles K. Atkin, "Mass Media Information Campaign Effectiveness," in Ronald E. Rice and William J.Paisley, eds., *Public Communication Campaigns* (Beverly Hills: Sage Publications, 1981), pp. 265-279 Quotation is on page 276.

[56] Richard E. Petty and John T. Cacioppo, *Attitudes and Persuasion: Classic and Contemporary Approaches* (Iowa: Wm. C. Brown, 1981) pp. 72-73.

[57] Note that legal consequences could still be discussed, as required by audit requirements

[58] Icek Ajzen and Martin Fishbein, *Understanding Attitudes and Predicting Social Behavior* (Englewood Cliffs, New Jersey: Prentice-Hall, Inc., 1980, p. 24.

[59] Howard Leventhal, Martin A. Safer, and Daphne M. Panagis, "The Impact of Communications on the Self-Regulation of Health Beliefs, Decisions and Behavior," *Health Education Quarterly*, Spring 1981. Also see James E. Maddux and Ronald W. Rogers, "Protection Motivation and Self-Efficacy: A Revised Theory of Fear Appeals and Attitude Change," *Journal of Experimental Social Psychology*, 1983, 19(5): 9. Also see Witte and Allen above.

[60] Stephen R. Sutton, "Fear-Arousing Communications: A Critical Examination of Theory and Research," in J. Richard Eiser, ed., *Social*

A sanitarian's attempt to show sympathy to site personnel, while potentially less stressful, might *not* produce public health improvements. Fear arousal is important in influencing the client's desire to change, even if the effect on actual behavior is indirect or inconsistent. It also sharpens the client's resolve to prepare themselves better to use the coping strategy. Bandura states that

> an aid to good performance is a strong sense of self-efficacy to withstand failures coupled with some uncertainty (construed in terms of the challenge of the task . . .) . . . to spur preparatory acquisition of knowledge and skills[61]

Thus, while few sanitarians relish the role of enforcer, some aspect of that role is essential to remind clients that compliance maintenance is a dynamic, on going task. A consistent enforcement protocol reminds clients that legal enforcement is an ever present, important resource.[62]

Fear arousal can have a negative effect, interfering with information processing.

This effect has already been implied above. A fear-arousing message without effective solutions[63] raises anxiety and may trigger relapse or regressive behaviors[64]. Resulting tensions and anxiety could slow any

---

Psychology and Behavioral Medicine (CITY: John Wiley & Sons, Ltd. 1982), pp. 303-325.

[61] Albert Bandura "Self Efficacy Mechanism in Human Agency" *American Psychologist* 1982 v. 37 (2) pp. 122-147 quote on p. 123

[62] Clients who see inconsistency here might use it to discredit the sanitarian and delay or avoid compliance.

[63] The client must perceive the solution as viable *and* effective to relieve their anxiety.

[64] R. F. Soames Job, PhD, "Effective and Ineffective Use of Fear in Health Promotion Campaigns," *American Journal of Public Health*, February 1988, 78(2): 163-167.

lasting behavioral change[65]. For example, a lengthy negative site report or one not accompanied by coping strategies, available resources or offers of sanitarian assistance might trigger helplessness, inactivity, or a defensive outburst. Dividing that evaluation into several site visits might produce more favorable results.

Fear arousal will be more effective when accompanied by viable solutions.

Fear arousal strengthens the client's attitudes about change and their *intention* to act; while this is a positive step, other factors (e.g., community support, self-efficacy, consultative and educational resources) motivate them to the actual *change* in behavior. While fear and anxiety may cause the client to listen to and process the message, whether or not they *accept* it or *act on it* are entirely different issues.

To motivate clients toward behavioral change, the sanitarian must clearly define (a) future consequences of noncompliance, positive as well as negative; and (b) standards against which future performance will be evaluated.

Helpful in this effort is modeling by a credible source as well as opportunity to practice the coping strategy. From Bandura . . .

> Until effective coping behaviors are developed, threats produce high emotional arousal and various defensive maneuvers[66] . . . (*and*) exposure to models performing feared activities without any harmful effects weakens defensive behavior, reduces fears and creates favorable changes in attitudes[67] . . . (*and*) anxiety arousal to threats is likewise diminished by modeling, and is even more thoroughly

---

[65] Albert Bandura, *Social Learning Theory* (New Jersey: Prentice-Hall, 1977), pp. 60-62. Fear arousal may exist coincidentally but does not *correlate* to message attention; effective coping strategies will resolve the anxiety.

[66] Albert Bandura, *Social Learning Theory*, (Englewood Cliffs, New Jersey: Prentice-Hall, Inc.) pp. 61-62.

[67] Albert Bandura, *Social Learning Theory* (Englewood Cliffs, New Jersey: Prentice-Hall, Inc. 1977) p.49

eliminated by experienced mastery achieved through participant modeling.[68]

Clients may be fearful about attempting some behaviors in the sanitarian's presence[69]. For this reason, modeling and reinforcing desired behaviors are important parts of a site evaluation. There is an inverse relationship between the client's fear and anxiety levels and their perceived self-efficacy regarding the coping strategy. As skills mastery and self-efficacy levels increase, fear and anxiety decrease; in contrast, lower perceived self-efficacy levels can elevate the individual's fear and anxiety to levels 'that far exceed the fear experienced during the actual threatening situation'[70]. Modeling and practice sessions, however time consuming, can greatly improve compliant behavior.[71]

There must be a clear link defined between the site evaluation report (documentation) and the desired end result (improved sanitation status, reduced public health risk, more favorable site reviews by the sanitarian). Otherwise, the site report becomes the focus of the site visit, not the means to a beneficial desired end result.

Coping strategies must have two parts: clearly defined outcomes (*goal specificity*) allow clients to regulate their own behavior; and achievable, realistic outcomes (*goal proximity*) may help clients to retain optimism. The client must perceive the end result as practical and effective in order to reduce anxiety and tension.

---

[68] Albert Bandura, "'Self-Efficacy: Toward a Unifying Theory of Behavioral Change" <u>Psychology Review</u>, 1977, 84(2): 191-215. Quote on page 199

[69] The author experienced this during a site evaluation. It was the lunch hour, the dining room was full of customers, yet no employees were in the kitchen. The kitchen employees were discovered huddled outside in the snow. The manager explained that they could not make mistakes if they were out of the kitchen!

[70] Albert Bandura, "Self-Efficacy: Toward a Unifying Theory of Behavioral Change" <u>Psychology Review</u>, 1977, 84(2): 191-215 p. 199

[71] Albert Bandura, "Self-Efficacy: Toward a Unifying Theory of Behavioral Change" <u>Psychology Review</u>, 1977, 84(2): 191-215—link of fear arousal and self-efficacy pp. 198-199

Since environmental health concerns often have a chronic or subclinical impact, strategies must have a compelling argument to be persuasive. If coping behaviors are not apparent or discussed during a site visit, and legal consequences of noncompliance are discussed, the client may experience panic or helplessness. If the anxiety is too great, the client will ignore or repress these solutions.

FEAR AROUSAL SUMMARY

Fear arousal and anxiety are difficult emotions for sanitarians to control during site visits, for both their clients and themselves. Clients already have some level of anxiety anticipating the inspection; the inspection incrementally adds to that. Sanitarians must work hard to diffuse these reactions and focus instead on the public health status of the facility. Current trends toward uniforms, badges, guns, and ticket writing only add to this anxiety while not increasing message credibility; the sanitarian's knowledge and persuasion increase the latter.

While fear and anxiety can be effective weapons to obtain the client's *attention* to difficult messages, behavioral change is driven by different factors. Since it is difficult to gauge the level of tension during a site inspection[72] and since the effects of fear arousal are not clear or uniform,[73] sanitarians should only expect a limited application of the concept; i.e., getting the client's attention. It may take several inspections to accurately gauge the client's state of mind and determine whether or not fear arousal is an appropriate tool to use. Once that is achieved, energies must focus on the presence and importance of coping strategies. All compliance strategies must be exhausted before turning to the use of fear arousal techniques.

Otherwise, two results are likely, both undesirable: (a) an inexperienced, less-confident client may be overcome, allowing their fear to "direct behavior in unwanted ways [and] arouse feelings of hopelessness or feelings that one

---

[72] An individual who initially seems antagonistic may actually be overwhelmed by other issues or amenable to the required changes in smaller doses. Appearances can be deceiving, especially during a stress-filled, pressured inspection. A shorter revisit might be in order to sort things out.

[73] Icek Ajzen and Martin Fishbein *Understanding and Predicting Social Behavior* (Englewood Cliffs, New Jersey: Prentice-Hall, Inc. 1980) p. 222 'The literature on communication and persuasion reveals virtually no consistent findings concerning the effects of any given manipulation on attitude change"

cannot cope . . ."[74][75]; or (b) a confident, experienced client may attempt to discredit the messenger (sanitarian) rather than deal with the message and change behaviors. In the latter case, the public health concern will become a political one, with the sanitarian, not sanitation, the problem.

One additional note about fear arousal concerns the client's required attendance at educational programs (e.g., food service certification). While a legal requirement compels the client's attendance to listen to the information, sanitarians should not expect a great deal beyond that. Other factors beyond fear arousal promote understanding, retention, and use of the information. Research on the effects of food service certification programs appears to support this statement.[76]

Suggestion for Sanitarians: When clients are angry or antagonistic during a site visit, sanitarians may be tempted to resort to high fear messages to assert their authority. It might be better, instead, to summarize the positive accomplishments from that date and schedule another site visit to revisit noncompliant issues. The client may need time to digest the information and site visit results: the return visit may show progress from this process.

---

[74] Howard Leventhal, Martin A. Safer, and Daphne M. Panagis, "The Impact of Communications on the Self-Regulation of Health Beliefs, Decisions and Behavior," *Health Education Quarterly*, Spring 1981, pp. 3-13.

[75] R. F. Soames Job, PhD, "Effective and Ineffective Use of Fear in Health Promotion Campaigns," *American Journal of Public Health*, February 1988, 78(2): 163-167.

[76] Jerry Wright, MPH, and Lindson Feun, PhD, "Food Service Manager Certification: An Evaluation of Its Impact," *National Journal of Environmental Health*, 49(1):12-15. In this study, increased inspection frequency had a statistically significant positive effect on sanitation in food service operations. Food service certification, however, did **not** correlate significantly with improved sanitation status.

CRITIQUE:
POOR DESIGN OF EDUCATION AND COMMUNICATION EFFORTS

One premise of this book is that the inspection based system negatively evaluates facilities and sites, creating dissonance without providing coping strategies. If coping strategies were explained and demonstrated for the client, cognitive dissonance might not be so traumatic. In rebuttal, sanitarians point to what they see as comprehensive[77] education and communication efforts. This, they feel, is evidence that clients have the needed information and resources to comply, if only they would take advantage of it.

There are training programs, publications, audio-visual materials and public relations campaigns offered at local sites such as libraries, schools and local government offices, often at nominal charge. These do provide people with the information and resources they need to comply. That much is true. In fact, compliant individuals appear to find the information and use it successfully. From this evidence comes the argument that compliance is practical and possible, if people are motivated *and* have the skills and resources with which to act. (Of course, this last factor is so often missing from most educational programs[78].)

Unfortunately, several errors in design and logic reduce the effect of these community outreach efforts. First and foremost, the educational design is based on the theory that, given the information, 'reasonable'

---

[77] This again points to most sanitarians' desire to work holistically and not merely to enforce.

[78] Goldsmith and Hochbaum (Francis J. Goldsmith, Godfrey M. Hochbaum, "Changing People's Behavior Toward the Environment," *Public Health Reports*, May-June 1975, 90(3): pp. 231-234.) rebut this point, saying, "too often we emphasize what people can do without informing them how they can do it" (p. 232). The poor design of education programs makes it difficult for clients to find the information and resources needed to change behaviors, even if they are actively seeking it.

people will figure out the rest of the process independently, i.e. find the needed resources and skills, apply the information and change behaviors. To the public health mentality, the process of behavioral change should be obvious. For that reason, public outreach efforts provide information and concept training, without any attempt to motivate or persuade clients to apply it. Retrospective motivation occurs in the form of fear arousal and legal enforcement.

There are good reasons for these omissions; in order to include discussion and demonstration of coping strategies, a portion of the program would need to occur at the facility site, to observe and motivate skills mastery. While this change is possible and practical, it would cost more in resources, for clients and sanitarians alike. When these costs are compared to the failures of traditional lecture formats, however, the changes seem worthwhile.

Education programs are presently designed using a three step, school-system format: classroom, lecture, and exam. Participants demonstrate "learning" based on their exam performance; food service managers, for example, are "certified" if they successfully complete an examination of food sanitation concepts. This is a major error in that some concepts must be mastered *entirely*, not merely enough to pass an examination. For example, it is clearly not acceptable if a participant becomes certified without knowing safe food temperatures, approved methods for hand washing, approved cleaning and sanitizing methods for utensils or food storage to avoid cross-contamination. These are major food safety concepts that every certified food service operator must know and be able to use competently: there is hardly enough time to consult a textbook during every sanitation crisis. Yet, a passing examination score of seventy-five percent is used to indicate evidence of operational expertise; it actually means the participant knows enough to answer three-quarters of the examination concepts. Would a food consumer be comfortable with these results, wondering which concepts are unfamiliar and possibly ill applied?.

National testing services argue that it would be impractical to administer an examination requiring successful completion of specific questions. In fact, a short quiz could be administered by the program instructor, before the participant is allowed to complete the national examination. While this might be inconvenient and would reduce the numbers of certified participants, it would lend more credibility to the label of 'certified operator'. At the present time, that label is used by entire industries to indicate someone knowledgeable and expert in the profession. In fact, they are knowledgeable in as little as three-quarters of the examination questions; since the use of the information is never evaluated, there is no way to know how expert they are in any aspect of the job[79].

Furthermore, the program design is based on a major misconception of human behavior and learning, the "fallacy of the empty vessel". It is assumed that food service managers arrive at the classroom *without* preconceived ideas about food service sanitation, an assumption far from the truth. The wide range of cultures and education levels in just the food service industry illustrate the error in this thinking. (The current 'solution' to this problem seems to be reprinting the same mistake in multiple languages.)

It is true that many other learning programs are designed using this format. All school system education is designed in this manner (it should be noted, however, that many schools have moved from lectures to open classroom and integrated disciplinary approaches.) However, while the design works well for children, for whom rote memorization drills are essential for a learning foundation, adults do not learn in this manner. Adults need a clearly defined application for the information they are learning, a behavior or skill they understand and feel confident they can perform. While information can be learned well enough to perform adequately on an examination, the key is whether it can be applied in the real world[80]. Fishbein and Ajzen comment on this fallacy, stating that

> researchers in the health domain often assume that the greater the accuracy of a person's information concerning a given illness or course of treatment, the more likely it is that the person will adopt appropriate health-protective behaviors. As

---

[79] Sanitarians know the answer, however, when, during site evaluations, they find the textbook hidden in a desk drawer and a lengthy, critical evaluation report on their laptop computer.

[80] Ironically, the efforts of some program designers to make education more tolerable with computer software, varied audio-visual materials and other types of entertainment only obscure the program objectives and applications.

reasonable as this may appear, the empirical evidence provides minimal support . . . [81]

If, in fact, the ultimate interest is applying the information and changing behaviors, different educational principles are needed for that criterion. Attendance and successful completion of an examination are only the first steps in the process.[82] Research shows, for instance, that the single most important factor influencing behavioral change is the participant's perceived self-efficacy. There are two phases to this concept: a belief about one's ability to act as recommended (self-efficacy) and a belief about the behavior's effectiveness (coping response efficacy).[83] Still, rather than evaluate the participants' skills mastery, health agencies continue to use attendance and examination scores as a measure of effective learning and program effectiveness.[84]

There are several reasons for this decision, aside form the obvious one of convenience. First, the classroom format is the most efficient use of time and resources to reach the widest range of people. An interactive, experientially based program, while most effective in promoting behavioral change, would require a sanitarian to either spend more time observing at the facility site or spend more money developing more complicated educational

---

[81] Martin Fishbein and Icek Ajzen, *Predicting and Changing Behavior: The Reasoned Action Approach* (New York: Psychology Press, 2010), p. 242.

[82] William McGuire, "Theoretical Foundations of Campaigns," in Ronald E. Rice and William J. Paisely, eds., *Public Communication Campaigns* (Beverly Hills, London: Sage, 1981), pp. 44-54. There are twelve conditional steps from the point of learning the information to behavioral change. "Since these probabilities tend to be considerably less than 1.00, their product is usually a quite small number" (51).

[83] Albert Bandura, *Social Learning Theory* (Englewood Cliffs, New Jersey: Prentice-Hall, 1977), p. 79; Irwin Rosenstock et al., "Social Learning Theory and the Health Belief Model," *Health Education Quarterly*, Summer 1988, 15(2): 175-180.

[84] A discussion of education program design follows below. One implication, however, is that one phase of program evaluation must occur during site evaluations, where client application of knowledge can be accurately reviewed.

media or learning modules. This could be disruptive to facility activities as well as to the health agency's budget. The decision to promote classroom formatted programs, however, severely restricts the program's effectiveness; *this* limitation must be taken into account when program effectiveness is evaluated. A second reason is more theoretical, based in psychodynamic reasoning. That theory implies that there is no purpose in prospective analysis or interventions to influence behavior: those explorations would be fruitless and yield no defined result. This applies first to inspections, where education and consultation tasks, central to interventions, gradually are distorted to be interrogative functions, and extends to education and training programs, where information is given through lecture, not discussion or discovery.[85]

The "fallacy of the empty vessel"[86] suggests that individuals come to an educational program with no preconceptions about the subject matter that might 'pollute' the learning process. Their minds are similar to empty 'vessels' ready to filled with knowledge. It is assumed that clients arrive at the learning experience with "blank slates" or "empty vessels" on which information will be "written" and applied.

Stephen Polgar discusses this concept in connection with the introduction of Western medicine into third-world societies (Mayan culture); in that earlier time, it was incorrectly assumed that the native ill population would welcome this assistance without preexisting attitudes and beliefs from their own culture. From these studies evolved the contemporary concept of an authoritarian Western physician, linked to the idea that individuals with illness symptoms ("sick role" patients) were expected to adopt the doctor's regimen and get "better." Polgar suggests that "change agents . . . often resort to the mass media for communicating new information and suppose that . . . they will effect the adoption of new health practices."[87]

---

[85] Albert Bandura, *Social Foundations of Thought & Action: A Social Cognitive Theory* (Englewood Cliffs, New Jersey: Prentice-Hall, 1986), pp. 2-4. (A critique of psychodynamic theory and psychological motivators.)

[86] Steven Polgar, "Health and Human Behavior: Areas of Interest Common to the Social and Medical Sciences" *Cultural Anthropology*, April 1962,. 3(2): 159-205.

[87] Steven Polgar, "Health and Human Behavior: Areas of Interest Common to the Social and Medical Sciences" *Cultural Anthropology*, April 1962,. 3(2) p. 176.

Sanitarians often find themselves proponents of this fallacy, believing, after years of familiarity with their work, that everyone else should be in ready agreement about its importance. Education program design echoes this thinking, in that there is a strong *presumed* link between presenting information and the participant's adoption of new sanitation behaviors. This is one reason why pre- and post-program needs assessment studies are rarely conducted; 'basic' information that everyone knows (or *should* know), e.g. how to mop a floor, wash their hands or use a food thermometer, is already assumed through theory. (Site evaluations show the opposite, more often than not.)

Reasonable people ('reasonable' from the sanitarian's perspective) *should* accept inspection reports (or education information) and act on them correctly. If they do not, no excuses are allowed; thus, rather than examine the educational program or sanitation system design for errors, the "victim" is "blamed" for his or her predicament. It is only a short leap in this logic toward applying examination scores as an indication of behavioral change; i.e., a passing score indicates improved sanitation status. (In fact, studies of environmental health programs rely on reasoning such as this.)[88]

Sanitarians and physicians, both trained in the sciences, view noncompliant people in this manner.[89] An ill person *ought* to follow the doctor's regimen and get better; this is a reasonable expectation for personal and public health and increased social productivity. Critiquing the regimen or the sanitarian's inspection report would be insulting and potentially professionally damaging; under the psychodynamic perspective, it should be enough for the sanitarian or physician to provide the information or describe the problem. A lecture, pamphlet,

---

[88] Jerry Wright, MPH, and Lindson Feun, PhD, "Food Service Manager Certification: An Evaluation of Its Impact," *National Journal of Environmental Health*, 49(1):12-15 is one of many examples. There are numerous studies where examination scores are used as a base for predicting successful facility operation

[89] Samuel Bloom and Robert Wilson, ""Patient-Practitioner Relationships," in Howard E. Freeman et al., eds., *Handbook of Medical Sociology*, 3rd ed. (Englewood Cliff, New Jersey: Prentice-Hall, Inc., 1963, 1972, 1979), pp. 275-296. For discussions of similarities of physicians and sanitarians, see Shattuck (footnote 108) (footnote 5).

newsletter, press release, or written report becomes the essence of public health communication and education efforts[90].

Polgar touches on this idea when he comments on the "somewhat authoritarian character" of "the health actor's relationship to the recipient in Western countries."[91]. Rosenstock comments that patients do not ask for clarification of regimens due to "the professional distance that the white-coated physician has been socialized to keep . . ."[92] It is not a far leap in logic to see sanitarians in an environmental "physician's" role, where they diagnose and prescribe environmental treatments.

In fact, effective educational program and inspection intervention designs *should* be extremely complicated procedures, singular and specific to the population, site, or facility.[93] There are numerous input and output variables that influence the likelihood of behavioral change, not merely the delivery of information. The recipient's prior knowledge and attitudes, potential barriers to change, and other environmental factors must be considered. *No prior knowledge can be assumed*[94], especially with the wide range of social and demographic variables found in program participants. Most messages must be repeated in different variations until the appropriate response is produced.[95]

---

[90] It came as quite a shock to the author when, upon entry to public health graduate studies in behavioral science, he was informed by a professor that handing out a pamphlet was not equivalent to health education.

[91] Steven Polgar, "Health and Human Behavior: Areas of Interest Common to the Social and Medical Sciences" *Cultural Anthropology*, April 1962,. 3(2: p. 177.

[92] Irwin M. Rosenstock, "Patients' Compliance with Health Regimens," *Journal of the American Medical Association*, 234(11/27/75): 402-403.

[93] The design of educational programs will be discussed later in this book. The point here is that current program design is ineffective and contrary to that recommended in the literature.

[94] An extremely important point: existing knowledge **must** be measured and verified, before it can be assumed in the program design. The costs of developing and presenting education programs, as well as the costs of inefficacious programs in noncompliant behavior both demand the use of needs assessments.

[95] William McGuire, "Theoretical Foundations of Campaigns," in Ronald E. Rice and William J. Paisely, eds., *Public Communication Campaigns* (Beverly

While this attention to detail makes program design more complicated, ignorance of it makes program evaluations and subsequent site evaluations more disappointing than needed.

In reality, adults "do not simply respond to stimuli; they *interpret* them"[96] based on existing attitudes and information. Adult learners do much more than respond to information; they act on it based on expectations formed before they enter the classroom or learning experience. (This is the foundation of educational behavioral objectives, a statement of program expectations for participants to consider prior to registration.) There is a dynamic interaction and influence between information, behavior, and environmental influences. This process must be anticipated and influenced by the instructor. What factors might influence a student's attitude toward the information? People

> are neither driven by inner forces nor buffeting by environmental stimuli . . . their decisions to act are tempered by thought processes, influenced by external forces but not overwhelmed by either . . . [Human behavior is] a continuous reciprocal interaction between cognitive, behavioral, and environmental determinants.[97]

Sanitarians may have two objections to this discussion: first, that many clients successfully complete these education programs and benefit from them; and second, that limited resources require the use of classroom teaching to distribute the information to as many clients as possible.

In the first instance, it is true that some clients do benefit; these individuals, however, since skills and coping strategies are usually not presented in these programs, these individuals must already have a

---

Hills, London: Sage, 1981), pp. 44-54.

[96] Albert Bandura, *Social Learning Theory* (Englewood Cliffs, New Jersey: Prentice-Hall, 1977), p. 59.

[97] Albert Bandura, *Social Foundations of Thought & Action: A Social Cognitive Theory* (Englewood Cliffs, New Jersey: Prentice-Hall, Inc. 1986), p. 12, and Albert Bandura, *Social Learning Theory,* (Englewood Cliffs, New Jersey: Prentice-Hall, Inc. 1977) pp. 11-12.

foundation in place (resources, skills, self-efficacy) with which to apply the information. There is also the question of whether or not they already knew the information and attended to please authority or would simply have obtained the information elsewhere[98]. While sanitarians have limited resources with which to present education programs, the program results must be viewed skeptically with these limitations in mind.

---

[98] The author's informal knowledge assessments during food service certification programs suggests that many participants were knowledgeable enough to pass the examination without attending the program.

CONSIDERING A NEW PARADIGM

The previous discussion stressed the inadequacy of the psychodynamic approach, the overreliance on the use of fear arousal for interventions, and the inadequate design of education programs. It was lengthy and comprehensive due to the deeply entrenched acceptance of psychodynamic theory and the existing inspection approach. (In fact, the solution sought by health professionals in the face of ineffectiveness has been, ironically, further reliance on the system; i.e., stronger enforcement actions!)

This book proposes a new intervention design based on current knowledge about decision-making processes. The objective is to integrate this design with the existing system and phase in changes incrementally. Research will be needed to determine its effectiveness and the most efficacious design. This is not, it must be emphasized, an attempt to rework the sanitarian's job or the nature of the profession; it only proposes a wider focus for understanding and influencing noncompliance, based on alternative explanations.

In seeking a new paradigm, it is important to first look at what is actually true, by research standards, about health behaviors and decision making. Then the Health Belief Model is applied to environmental health concerns, with consideration of Social Learning Theory concepts. The intent is not to propose a new model but rather to establish guidelines for sanitarians to use in evaluating the presence of noncompliant behavior.

Health behavior and decision making are rational processes.

"[H]uman beings are usually quite rational and make systematic use of the information available to them."[99] "People are motivated to hold correct attitudes . . ."[100] This means that "people use whatever information

---

[99] Icek Ajzen and Martin Fishbein, *Understanding Attitudes and Predicting Social Behavior* (Englewood Cliffs, New Jersey: Prentice-Hall, Inc., 1980), p. 24.

[100] Richard E. Petty and John T. Cacioppo, *Communication and Persuasion: Central and Peripheral Routes to Attitude Change* (New York: Springer-Verlag, 1986), p. 6.

is available to them in a reasonable fashion to arrive at a behavioral decision."[101] It *does not* mean they always arrive at the *correct* conclusions, however.

These statements are really the underpinning of a new intervention paradigm. The present assumption about noncompliant clients is that they have the required information and resources available but choose to ignore or misuse them. The above statement suggests this might not be the case; while the client acts incorrectly, they act rationally based on the information they have available, albeit it limited or biased.[102]

Adults do not experiment with behaviors; they carefully consider their actions, gathering information, observing other situations, and rehearsing their plan of action. Thus, aside from medical anomalies, people usually have a reason behind their actions, however eccentric it may seem. Of course, individuals have different priorities, and that is the challenge of analyzing noncompliance. Still, the outcome is more predictable than that implied by psychodynamic theory or by the experience of stressful fast-paced inspections. Patient sanitarians will find this rational thought process emerging over the course of their site visits.

This discussion suggests several conclusions: first, given persistence and patience, the sanitarian will eventually[103] provide the proper mix of information and skills modeling to bring the client to comply; second, despite superficial impressions from one or two site visits, clients may actually be attempting to move toward change, however subtle the process; third, the sanitarian's use of legal enforcement may occur too early in present interventions, choking off efforts toward compliance; and fourth, a proactive paradigm to encourage the client's efforts may in some cases yield success.

---

[101] Martin Fishbein, "A Reasoned Action Approach," in Icek Ajzen et al., eds., *Prediction and Change of Health Behavior: Applying the Reasoned Action Approach* (New Jersey: Erlbaum Associates, 2007), p. 282. This implies the importance of complete accurate information and the availability of resources.

[102] Implying the need to use a network to distribute correct information to clients.

[103] It cannot be emphasized enough, that patience may not always be possible and excuses for noncompliance cannot always be tolerated. Imminent hazards must be abated quickly.

This is not an excuse for inactivity, however. Bandura notes that excuses cannot be used to mask 'weak programs' or the absence of 'environments conducive for learning'. Sometimes, patience is not good enough; 'for many, it turns out to be a long wait'[104].

Behaviors are driven by motivators unique to each person.

Causality is unique to each individual and is not precisely predictable. The positive aspect here is that intervention is not limited to enforcement and fear arousal; the system must expand to adequately deal with as many noncompliance cases as possible. In the case of persistent noncompliance, sanitarians can look to other factors besides the success or failure of legal enforcement. Individuals are no more motivated by recalcitrance, greed, and selfishness than they are by legal threats, personal anxieties, or the Golden Rule. While it is not possible to predict a client's reaction prospectively, it *is* possible to predict the evaluative processes clients undergo prior to behavioral change.

The individual's stated intention to act is a good predictor of further actions.

An individual forms an intention to act based on his or her attitudes and beliefs about the change. The intention to act has a strong correlation to the change in behavior, but only if the precise type and the precise time period are specified[105]; one study shows significant correlations between

---

[104] Albert Bandura, *Social Learning Theory* (Englewood Cliffs, New Jersey: Prentice-Hall, Inc. 1977) p. 183

[105] Richard E. Petty and John T. Cacioppo, *Attitudes and Persuasion: Classic and Contemporary Approaches* (Iowa: Wm. C. Brown, 1981 (correlation estimates), pp. 198-199; Martin Fishbein and Icek Ajzen, Martin Fishbein and Icek Ajzen, *Predicting and Changing Behavior: The Reasoned Action Approach* (New York: Psychology Press, 2010), pp. 43, 53-73; Albert Bandura, *Social Learning Theory* (Englewood Cliffs, New Jersey: Prentice-Hall, Inc. 1977), p. 162.

intentions and actual behavior ranging from 0.69 to 0.90.[106] The accuracy of these figures, however, depends on how precisely intentions are stated and measured, in terms of the specific behavior (washing hands properly versus washing hands using soap, hot water, and scrubbing for twenty seconds) and time frame (today, the next ninety days, the next year).

The extent of knowledge about the client's attitudes and beliefs will influence the final intervention design.[107] The client's spoken or written intention to change behaviors is vital, as it is with any type of social contract. This can be attained through a verbal interview (i.e. 'How likely is it that you can train your employees in this behavior in the next 30 days?') but the preferred method is to have the individual sign a paper to indicate their commitment. (Legal conferences or hearings with noncompliant individuals often require "plans of action" to address noncompliance; in food sanitation, these may be HACCP ["hazard analysis and critical control points": a risk analysis and control plan] plans, standard operating procedures, or risk assessment reports completed and signed by the client.) The commitment could be in the form of a signature receiving the site evaluation report (i.e. the report might state that 'the person in charge, by their signature, states their intention to train employees to apply coping strategy X in the next 30 (thirty) days') or it might be a signed and dated written plan of action.

The individual's written commitment is an essential step toward behavioral change. Entry and exit interviews during site visits and conferences, however brief, are also important assessment tools. Feedback is very important to an accurate assessment. These interviews serve to draw out the client's beliefs and attitudes and, in turn, assess their intentions to act.[108]

---

[106] Icek Ajzen, "From Intentions to Actions," Ch. 5 in *Attitudes, Personality and Behavior*, 2nd ed. (Berkshire, England, and New York: Open University Press, McGraw-Hill, 2005) p. 99-116, more specifically pp. 100-103.

[107] Martin Fishbein and Icek Ajzen *Belief, Attitude, Intention and Behavior: An Introduction to Theory and Research* (Massachusetts: Addison-Wesley, 1975), pp. 8-18. Attitudes and beliefs referenced to action and behavioral change.

[108] Martin Fishbein and Icek Ajzen, *Predicting and Changing Behavior: The Reasoned Action Approach* (New York: Psychology Press, 2010), pp. 314-315. Correlation of stated intentions and actual behavior.

Behavioral change depends on factors in addition to the stated intention to act.

"Although people want to hold correct attitudes, the amount and nature . . . in which they are willing or able to engage . . . vary with individual and situational factors."[109] While a stated intention to act is a good clue to future types of behavior, *actual* behavior depends on specificity of intent, in both time frame and type of behavior ("Do you intend, in *x* days to avoid *y* problem by adopting *z* behaviors?" as opposed to "do you intend to do something soon about this problem?"), the stability of that intent, and the degree to which execution of the behavior is under the client's control.[110] The sanitarian may need to ask specific questions about the individual's strategy and time line for compliance.

The client's perceived self-efficacy or volitional (situational) control is an important factor. An individual may have a high level of perceived self-efficacy but not be confident of his or her continued *control* of the situation. There may be barriers in the form of a change-resistant absentee owner or a fluctuating money flow that restricts training opportunities. In other situations, the individual may understate their perceived self-efficacy in the presence of an authority figure. Others besides the person in charge, e.g. an experienced employee or an absentee owner, may actually be the authority figure and control facility operations. Thus an individual's perspective on compliance and their perceived self-efficacy expressed during an interview might not directly correlate with reality. It may take the sanitarian several site visits and some time observing facility operations to gain a reasonable assessment of the situation.

---

[109] Richard E. Petty and John T. Cacioppo, *Communication and Persuasion: Central and Peripheral Routes to Attitude Change* (New York: Springer-Verlag, 1986), p. 6.

[110] Martin Fishbein and Icek Ajzen *Belief, Attitude, Intention and Behavior: An Introduction to Theory and Research* (Massachusetts: Addison-Wesley, 1975), pp. 368-372; Icek Ajzen, *Attitudes, Personality and Behavior* (Berkshire, England, and New York: Open University Press, McGraw-Hill, 2005) pp. 100-116.

The sanitarian's clear communication of requirements and compliance dates, as well as modeling of skills, in conjunction with timely inspections and consistent enforcement, will give clients a consistent benchmark of expectations.[111][112] This, in turn, may help the client's motivation to act as well as their perceived self-efficacy.

Some clients are beyond the reach of any intervention.

Despite all attempts at persuasion, some people will never comply; the public health risk they create must be abated as quickly as possible. Other individuals would like to comply but, for whatever reason, are not ready or prepared to do so. Stage theorists suggest that the latter group lack "cognitive (or behavioral) readiness," and regardless of the intervention design and intensity (legal threats, education, or trilateral combinations), their actions eventually become compliant when they are ready. While sanitarians ideally should spend more time understanding the client's stages to action, emphasizing persuasive communication, they also must be able to recognize its limits and use legal enforcement readily and decisively. The presence of enforcement is vital to abate imminent short-term public health concerns, but, even if not used, its implied presence heightens the client's awareness of the sanitarian's message. Imminent health hazards must be abated: it may not always be possible to wait for the opportune psychologically positive moment.[113][114]

---

[111] Albert Bandura, *Social Learning Theory* (Englewood Cliffs, New Jersey: Prentice-Hall, 1977), p. 167.

[112] Jerry Wright, MPH, and Lindson Feun, PhD, "Food Service Manager Certification: An Evaluation of Its Impact," *National Journal of Environmental Health*, 49(1):12-15. In this study, increased inspection frequency had a statistically significant positive effect on sanitation in food service operations.

[113] Albert Bandura, *Social Learning Theory*, (Englewood Cliffs, New Jersey: Prentice-Hall, Inc. 1977) p. 183.

[114] Karen Glanz, Barbara K. Rimer, and Frances Marcus Lewis, eds., *Health Behavior and Health Education: Theory, Research and Practice*, 3rd ed. (San Francisco: John Wiley & Sons, 2002), pp.122-124.

SECTION SUMMARY: LEARNING PRINCIPLES

The preceding paragraphs suggest the following: first, given persistence and networking help, the client will eventually attain the needed information, attitudes, and skills to reach compliance; second, despite negative inspection results, clients may actually be moving toward compliance (there may be positive trends not measurable by the inspection); third, legal enforcement may be used too early, choking off those efforts; and fourth, a proactive paradigm to encourage the client's effort to comply may, in some cases, yield success where fear arousal and legal enforcement have failed.

THE HEALTH BELIEF MODEL[115]

Progressing Toward a Solution

Having discussed general decision-making concepts and recognizing the limits of the unilateral legal enforcement model, we look now at a structure for understanding environmental compliance and for instituting a public health network for change. The attempt here is not to propose a new behavioral model but to suggest a framework for analyzing noncompliance when it persists.

Health educators and behavioral scientists have developed many useful models for analyzing why clients reject recommendations for personal preventative health change (e.g., smoking cessation, weight loss, dental hygiene). This book proposes applying one of these models, the Health Belief Model (hereafter the Model), to environmental health decision making. The concepts in the Model should be addressed by sanitarians during any site evaluation and within any effective compliance intervention.

First, the Model and its factors are described; then the steps to developing an intervention strategy are outlined, along with

---

[115] Four resources were drawn upon for this discussion of the Health Belief Model, its components and applications: (1) Irwin M. Rosenstock, PhD, "Historical Origins of the Health Belief Model" *in* Marshall H. Becker, Ph.D., M.P.H, ed. *The Health Belief Model and Personal Health Behavior* (Thorofare, New Jersey: Charles B. Slack, Inc. 1974) pp. 1-8 (reprint of *Health Education Monographs* (1974) 2)—figure 3 is adapted from pg. 7; (2) Irwin M. Rosenstock, PhD, "The Health Belief Model and Preventive Health Behavior" in the same publication pp. 27-59; (3) MH Becker ed. "The Health Belief Model and Personal Health Behavior" in *Health Education Monographs (1974) 2:324-508* (the entire publication is devoted to the Model and its components): also (4) Karen Glanz, Barbara K. Rimer, and Frances Marcus Lewis, eds. *Health Behavior and Health Education: Theory, Research and Practice*, 3rd ed. (San Francisco: John Wiley & Sons, 2002), p. 45-52

recommendations for using the Model and other behavioral science concepts, in site evaluations.

Origins and Summary

The Model[116] was developed to explain why clients reject[117] recommendations to change personal preventative health behaviors. Early research concentrated on the failure to obtain health assessments (tuberculosis screening) and immunizations, followed by studies of personal health behaviors such as smoking cessation and weight control. Figure 3 shows the Model as it was originally proposed.

Using this Model, a health behavior change is evaluated in the context of the following areas of concern: perceived problem severity and susceptibility; perceived benefits of medical or therapeutic intervention; perceived benefits of the coping strategy; and patient knowledge of the condition and prescribed regimen.[118] The individual must have strong positive perceptions to consider a change in behavior. All concerns may not be processed concurrently or in the order stated in the Model. Some may receive ongoing review before, during, and after a crisis or concern.

---

[116] Discussed in website paper "HBM Interactive Outline," Kelli McCormarck Brown, University of South Florida, revision 1/11/99; Irwin Rosenstock's unpublished research grant summary of the similarities between social learning theory and the Health Belief Model (approximate date 1987-88; discussion in seminar attended by the author); Karen Glanz, Barbara K. Rimer, and Frances Marcus Lewis, eds. *Health Behavior and Health Education: Theory, Research and Practice*, 3rd ed. (San Francisco: John Wiley & Sons, 2002), pp. 45-63.

[117] Irwin M. Rosenstock 'Historical Origins of the Health Belief Model' in Marshall H. Becker, Ph.D., M.P.H, ed. *The Health Belief Model and Personal Health Behavior* (Thorofare, New Jersey: Charles B. Slack, Inc. 1974) pp. 7-8. The Model "had a clearcut avoidance orientation" in explaining why people avoid health conditions. Why they might adopt preventive positive health actions or how a positive health campaign might be designed are different matters.

[118] Irwin M. Rosenstock, PhD, "Patients' Compliance With Health Regimens," *Journal of the American Medical Association*, 11/27/1975, 234(4): 402-403.

For instance, a client *anticipating* the sanitarian's inspection might be concerned about their ability to comply, to fulfill the coping strategy, long before the actual site visit.

The Model was originally developed to analyze compliance with personal preventative health recommendations; however, it has been revised numerous times for use with more complicated environmentally based chronic illness conditions (more on this later).

Figure 3 divides the five areas of concern into three categories: individual perceptions, modifying factors, and likelihood of action. The individual's consideration of the problem's immediacy and severity, modified by prior knowledge, experience, and environmental pressures, creates a perception of the condition's threat. Consideration of perceived costs and benefits of taking action allow formation of an intention to act (Likelihood of Behavioral Change). The arrows in the graphic indicate how the factors influence each other: prior knowledge and socio-demographic data, for instance, influence cost-benefit considerations as well as the formation of the threat of condition. (There are reciprocal influences throughout, emphasizing the dynamics of decision-making processes.)

The Model is proposed here only as a situation-dependent framework for considering the reasons for environmental noncompliance. Sanitarians can look to these factors when noncompliance persists. There are numerous other theories from behavioral scientists that could easily have been used as examples; ideas from them are included in this book. In the succeeding pages, we look at ways sanitarians can use the Model's factors to make site evaluations easier to conduct and more efficacious. While the five factors are described in an organized progression, clients may not consider them in that order.

I. Individual perceptions[119]—susceptibility and severity (figure 3—first column). The client (manager or person in charge) must perceive that both[120] themselves *and* the facility are vulnerable to the

---

[119] The client's *perceptions*, not always reality, drive the final decision to act.

[120] One factor is whether the client's personal perceptions of susceptibility will apply as strongly to a facility or site for which they are responsible. There should be a good but not perfect correlation; most clients have a personal

condition (e.g., food-related illness) *and* that "the future occurrence of a given [condition] would have serious impact . . ."[121] The cited violation or concern must be perceived as strongly related to a serious and immediate condition.

One validity issue is whether the client's *personal* perceptions of susceptibility will apply as strongly to a community or public setting. Since there are multiple stakeholders and differing levels of interest in the facility (manager, owner), the correlation clearly will not be perfect. The author's field experience suggests, however, that the link will be strong: most clients, regardless of interest or stake, have a personal interest in the environmental concerns under evaluation. In other words, they eat food, swim, dispose of refuse or wastewater, and engage in environmentally sensitive activities; their corporate and personal activities interrelate. The strength of correlation will depend on the individual's control within the facility. In situations where there is a motivated person in charge but intermittent, difficult compliance, sanitarians may need to assess the importance of this factor.

Clients will already have a general perception of the general problem (environmental risk factors and related violations) and the threat posed by it prior to the sanitarian's arrival. These perceptions will be both *general* (anxiety over an approaching inspection and potential requirements) and *specific* (noncompliant conditions at the site may not yet have been resolved; the strategy for doing so may be unclear). In essence, they will have formed attitudes about how they will receive and process the information.

Perceptions of the problem's *susceptibility* (how immediate is it for the facility or the client?) and *severity* (if affected, how severe would be the impact?) will evolve throughout the site evaluation, relative to the report. One confounding problem may be an overemphasis on the facility's legal status and not on the public health condition. Many clients correlate their facility's sanitation status with the content of the evaluation report; i.e., if the report does not state it, it is not a concern. While this cannot

---

interest in the environmental concerns, and often they have a controlling interest in the site or facility.

[121] Irwin W. Rosentock, PhD, "Patients' Compliance with Health Regimens," *Journal of the American Medical Association*, 10/27/1975, 234(4): 402-403.

be avoided in some instances, too much emphasis is counterproductive and must be balanced. Sanitarians must continually direct attention to the site's overall public health status, not the report's length or number of violations cited. Part of this discussion might center around trends, positive or negative, leading toward or away from sanitation concerns.

Suggestions for Sanitarians[122]

Most clients probably have a clear idea that there are problems and consequences, *of some sort,* linked to the sanitarian's arrival on site. The sanitarian's first concern must be to be sure the client's perceptions are related to a public health concern not a political one. In other words, the client could easily perceive the sanitarian's legal presence as the main problem, not the prevention of illness or contagion. In that regard, the following are actions to consider:

- ✓ **Emphasize public health implications**—use newsletters, media releases and pamphlets to describe the potential public health impact of problems on that site visit. The Morbidity and Mortality Weekly Report (Centers for Disease Control), journals from environmental health related associations, journals from professional vocational groups (restaurants, water well drillers, swimming pool supply and water treatment, wastewater disposal and the like) and internet sites from the same groups often have case studies and research illustrating how imminent or critical violations can cause public health problems;

- ✓ **Be certain that site personnel observe the problem** as it occurs—While many sanitarians dislike having site personnel accompany them during the site evaluation, viewing the violation concurrently clarifies its importance and leaves no room for dispute. (This issue can be made positive by acknowledging the client's ownership of their facility). If clients do not accompany the sanitarian, they will either discount a problem's importance or insist on seeing it for themselves (at that time, the concern

---

[122] See the Appendix for more ideas.

may have been corrected, allowing the client to question its validity);

- ✓ **Deliver a credible message**—Provide the client with the most accurate, up to date message possible. Subscribe to technical journals, local newspapers and professional mailings (e.g. Morbidity and Mortality Weekly Report from the Centers for Disease Control), attend training programs and seminars and stay current on all recent professional developments. Talk to other sanitarians to learn effective ways to evaluate a facility and to write a site report.

The second concern will be to carefully gauge the level of fear arousal and not let this slow progress toward compliance.

- ✓ **Interact with clients** to determine their response to the site evaluation and their attitudes about the public health concerns just documented. This will give the sanitarian a gauge of the client's anxiety and resistance to change. Preferably this means a post evaluation interview but, if time is short, interact during the evaluation itself or schedule another short visit over a cup of coffee;

- ✓ **Use public health networking** to reinforce public health concerns as well as to supplement the sanitarian's credibility. The use of networking will be vital throughout in establishing an effective intervention.

II. Modifying factors (fig. 3, middle column). This group of factors is composed of (a) knowledge of the condition, (b) knowledge of the regimen (environmental influences), and (c) cues to action. [Note: suggestions from Section I above carry over to this section.]

The individual's processing of the message in step 1 produces both a perceived threat of the condition and some general intention to act (hopefully according to the sanitarian's wishes!) This perception will be influenced by environmental factors (socio-demographics, experience, education, prior knowledge), for both the individual (micro-) and the community (macro-),[123] as well as by cues from external and internal sources. The client's perceptions will also be modified by experience, education, and socio-demographic backgrounds (see the box in figure 3 "Age, Sex, Culture, Personality, Knowledge, Socioeconomics"). Development of perceptions will continue for some time after the initial site evaluation and may have changed by the time of the next meeting with the sanitarian.[124] Industry wide information, attitudes, and capital growth on a *community* level will influence decision making in the same way as the *individual's* capital growth, education, and attitudes. Input may be gathered from friends in the industry, professional associations, and the family, and it will be influenced by existing cultural and social factors, attitudes, and beliefs. There will be a reciprocal relationship between individual and environmental determinants,[125] suggesting that interventions must be conducted on both a macro- (community or networking) and micro- (personal, site evaluation) scale.

The individual's knowledge of the condition and prescribed change requirements is an important consideration. Biased information from other professional associates ('other sanitarians do not cite that item', 'no harm has come to restaurant *x* from that condition') or from personal sources (misconceptions such as 'hot food will sour if cooled too rapidly' or 'this family recipe will not taste right prepared by modern methods') can slow progress toward compliance.

While the sanitarian's primary reference is the site manager or person in charge, there will be a reciprocal influence between multiple stakeholders on-site (owner, employees, other managers), as well as between the sanitarian, site personnel, and other government officials (fire marshal, building officials, code enforcement personnel, insurance agents, and others). Government officials such as fire marshals and code enforcement inspectors will also be important; these individuals may enforce requirements contrary to health codes. Networking may be

---

[123] Martin Fishbein and Icek Ajzen, *Predicting and Changing Behavior: The Reasoned Action Approach* (New York: Psychology Press, 2010), p. 251.

[124] A constant theme in this book is that compliance cannot be attained through a single interaction or a single variable.

[125] Albert Bandura, *Social Learning Theory* (Englewood Cliffs, New Jersey: Prentice-Hall, 1977), p. 11-12.

needed to correct that information or find a common ground to satisfy both sets of codes. Employee attitudes also will significantly influence compliance; well-trained employees pressure others into compliance.

The individual's motivation to change will be pushed forward by legal implications, experiences of professional associates, media reports of related problems, and the like (see box 'Cues to Action-Legal, Media'). Research has shown that persistent repeat site visits and gradual, realistic, phased changes are positively correlated with increased sanitation status.[126] The sanitarian's ability to produce a persuasive message will also be vital; see the section on communications.

Cues, 'strategies to activate one's readiness,'[127] provide a critical push to action, influencing the importance of the first two factors (problem susceptibility and severity) in the Model. Cues become critical when the individual's motivation is weak or the sanitarian's message is not convincing on its own merits.[128] The sanitarian's influence (legal authority) might be the first factor in mind; however, other *external* cues include social pressures regarding the activity[129] (cohort groups such as family, friends, church groups, and professional groups who believe the change is important), media events (restaurant reviews, reports of foodborne illness), legal pressures, and, on the positive side, reinforcement from credible models and significant others (such as the sanitarian during the inspection or children who relate a school curriculum module about proper hand washing). *Internal* cues include the client's personal experience with the problem, such as illness after

---

[126] Jerry Wright, MPH, and Lindson Feun, PhD, "Food Service Manager Certification: An Evaluation of Its Impact," *National Journal of Environmental Health*, 1986, 49(1): 12-15. In this study, increased inspection frequency had a positive effect on sanitation in food service operations.

[127] Karen Glanz, Barbara K. Rimer and Frances Marcus Lewis, eds. *Health Behavior and Health Education*, p. 49 (chart used in figure 6; p. 52 (graphic used in figure 3)

[128] Elements of message *delivery* will be discussed later.

[129] Icek Ajzen and Martin Fishbein, "Introduction: A Theory of Reasoned Action," *Understanding Attitudes and Predicting Social Behavior* (Englewood Cliffs, New Jersey: Prentice-Hall, Inc., 1980), pp. 4-9.

eating at a restaurant or observing overt (aesthetically unpleasant!) critical violations during food preparation.

The sanitarian's influence, be it overt through inspections or simply implied by a neighborhood presence or a newsletter, is an essential external cue to remind the manager of the importance of change (and the legal consequences of inactivity). A sanitarian's inconsistency (inaccurate reporting, failure to take legal action) would give the client variable or false expectations and might delay or halt compliance. As was discussed in the section on fear arousal, it is important not to overemphasize these factors, especially to a client who already has formed strong positive attitudes of their importance. However, this can easily be overdone; any reminders of legal consequences should be paired with equal reminders of public health significance.

Site personnel may perceive cues as stressors and cease further activity. Thus cues must include both positive (recognition for achievement, license cost reduction) and negative (legal action, increased site visits) motivators, referencing resources, skills, and potential solutions. Modeling of correct behaviors, either by the sanitarian or respected employees, is an important positive cue to action. If this occurs in a neutral environment, without criticism, clients will be motivated to practice these behaviors afterwards. As a result, "exposure to models performing feared activities without any harmful effects weakens defensive behavior, reduces fears, and creates favorable changes in attitudes."[130]

If the problem is perceived to be imminent *and* serious, the individual will form an intention to act, *in some undefined manner*.[131] New information and/or observations create tension and anxiety; a decision to act is made to reduce this anxiety. A violation written for the first time, while received and considered, will probably not result in immediate compliance, due to a lag in developing perceptions and attitudes in response. This apparent lack of impact might be due to the lack of customer feedback about the concern, inconsistency in previous

---

[130] Albert Bandura, *Social Learning Theory* (Englewood Cliffs, New Jersey: Prentice-Hall, 1977) p. 49.

[131] More specifics will evolve with consideration of the remaining factors in the Model.

reports, resistance due to misinformation, cultural bias, or experience in the industry without any similar problems. The sanitarian should wait before attaching importance to this hesitation.

Patience and persistence will be needed to communicate the problem and solution, clearly and credibly. An educated, experienced individual may understand the problem well but discount its severity: their action may be delayed. Legal implications of noncompliance or other cues to action may need to be mentioned. In contrast, an inexperienced, less-educated manager will likely view the same violation more seriously, particularly when the message is delivered by a credible source and there are no contrary opinions or information. This individual may want to discuss coping strategies immediately. Fear arousal will need to be downplayed in this case, as too high a level may frighten the individual into inactivity. If the level of fear and tension is too high, there may be an attempt to redefine the problem as the fault of an overzealous sanitarian, not a public health issue.[132]

Suggestions for Sanitarians[133]

The suggestions for section I (networking, credibility, interviews) carry over to this section. The sanitarian's message must be persuasive enough to counter the client's misleading perceptions generated from his or her socio-demographic and cultural background and, most important, generated from dissonance. The ability to institute cues, legal action, must be visible and persuasive to the client but use should be reserved until *after* interviews with the client.

- ✓ **Emphasize public health implications**—use newsletters, media releases and pamphlets to describe the potential public health impact of problems on that site visit. The Morbidity and Mortality Weekly Report (Centers for Disease Control) often

---

[132] Stephen R. Sutton, "Fear-Arousing Communications: A Critical Examination of Theory and Research," in J. Richard Eiser, ed., *Social Psychology and Behavioral Medicine* (Hoboken, New Jersey: John Wiley & Sons, Ltd., 1982), pp. 303-325.

[133] See the Appendix for more ideas.

has case studies where imminent or critical violations caused an illness or outbreak;

- ✓ **Be certain that site personnel observe the problem** as it occurs—While many sanitarians dislike having site personnel accompany them during the site evaluation, viewing the violation together asserts its public health significance. If clients do not observe the problem, they will either discount its importance or insist on seeing it for themselves.

III. **Perceptions of the change**—("cost-benefit" balance; box in figure 3 titled "Perceived Benefits Versus Costs (Barriers)"). After forming an intention to act, the client will review and evaluate the costs and benefits of the *recommended* change. The strength of commitment will relate to the strength of the perceptions in step 1 ("Individual perceptions"). The sanitarian must provide a convincing coping strategy, well defined and modeled, in order to keep the client focused on the desired behavioral change. Otherwise the client will create a change more to their liking.

The client must perceive the coping strategy as *both* practical and effective, a good fit with available skills, training, and resources. For example, in order to hold safe food temperatures, is it best to spend money on repairing the refrigerator, buying a new thermometer, discarding the food after two hours, purchasing dry or crushed ice, training the staff, or a combination thereof? Each facility will have different resources and different needs.

The sanitarian must walk the individual through problem analysis, looking at a variety of possible solutions and offering training and resources where there are perceived barriers to action. Otherwise, a person who feels pressured to act, *without options*, will attempt to discredit the message and solution as impractical, ineffective, or expensive. For example, holding food at safe temperatures may be accomplished with little expense but will require extensive training and monitoring. Individuals apprehensive of staff training (many are well informed but afraid of public speaking!) may redefine the change as prohibitive, emphasizing expensive equipment replacement when their worry *should* be about conducting the training program. In this case, the sanitarian must assist with the training effort, perhaps by assisting with the first staff training or by providing notes on training techniques. In other instances, site personnel well versed in training may have trouble finding the money to purchase or repair equipment. The sanitarian's job will be different in that case. Sanitarians must spend some time sorting out costs and barriers to action during their evaluation interviews.

Often, one sanitation concern or violation carries a number of possible coping strategies, as well as associated costs. Costs might include equipment maintenance (refrigerators, ovens, and holding equipment), employee training, and temperature checks; benefits might be reduced insurance costs, improved employee morale, less food spoilage, avoidance of customer illness, and increased return business. While costs are inevitable, perceptions about them will provide a framework for influencing and understanding the noncompliance.

The client must perceive any barriers to change as surmountable. To some extent, barriers are linked to cost-benefit analysis (staff training carries a cost of time and skills but is also a barrier; apprehension of public speaking) but may extend beyond that point. A wide range of factors influence perceived barriers: these include financial costs, negative emotional reactions (painful, difficult, upsetting) to anticipated change, physical barriers (inconvenient, time-consuming), side effects or

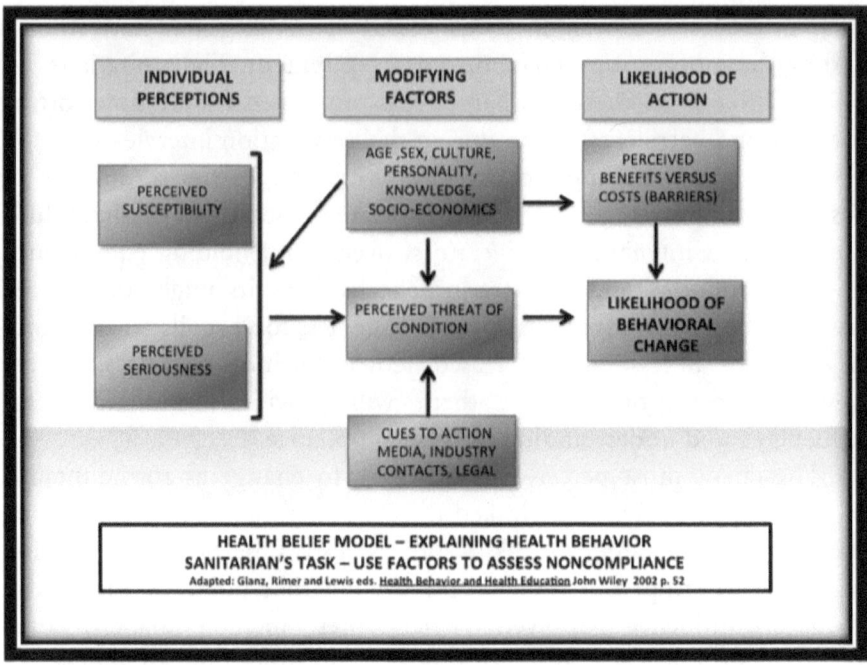

FIGURE 3: THE HEALTH BELIEF MODEL
Sources: Karen Glanz, Barbara K. Rimer and Frances Marcus Lewis, eds. *Health Behavior and Health Education: Theory, Research and Practice* 3rd Edition (San Francisco, California: Jossey-Bass 2002) p. 52; Irwin M. Rosenstock "Historical Origins of the Health Belief Model" *in* Marshall H. Becker, Ph.D., M.P.H, ed. *The Health Belief Model and Personal Health Behavior* (Thorofare, New Jersey: Charles B. Slack, Inc. 1974) p. 7)

repercussions of change, language translation, handicap access, accessibility factors, and personal characteristics.[134]

The *sanitarian* may be seen as a barrier to change if no positive changes in facility status are ever acknowledged and communication is always unilateral. Other barrier questions might center on the availability of resources (money for equipment, time to train employees) to get the job done.

A marginal cost-benefit analysis (i.e. either negative or not convincingly positive) may result in cognitive dissonance, a conflict between what is clearly a pressing problem[135] (the first two factors have already been acknowledged) and costs that seem prohibitive. Sanitarians must discuss barriers mentioned by clients, along with solutions, in order to gauge their importance as well as to plan interventions. As with other factors above, success at this stage will depend on the strength of earlier responses.

Suggestions for Sanitarians[136]

At this stage, the client has formed an indistinct intention to take action and is reviewed coping strategies. It is up to the sanitarian to make the desired coping strategy attractive and practical. The client must see that strategy as effective (it will resolve the problem) and efficacious (it is practical and within the client's abilities and resources).

---

[134] Nancy Janz, Victoria L. Champion, and Victor J. Strecher, *The Health Belief Model*, in Karen Glanz, Barbara K. Rimer, and Frances Marcus Lewis, eds., *Health Behavior and Health Education: Theory, Research and Practice*, 3rd ed. (San Francisco: John Wiley & Sons, 2002) pp. 45-66. Also see Irwin M. Rosenstock, PhD, Victor J. Strecher, PhD, MPH, and Marshall H. Becker, PhD, MPH, "Social Learning Theory and the Health Belief Model," *Health Education Quarterly*, (Summer 1988), 15(2): 175-183.

[135] In this case, the client has already acknowledged the importance of the Model's first two factors or he or she would not still be considering the change.

[136] See the Appendix for more ideas.

A large part of this section concerns perceived self-efficacy. A great number of suggestions are offered in that section. The sanitarian, however, can help to make the coping strategy appear more practical.

- ✓ **Illustrate how the coping strategy works**—list area facilities presently using the coping strategy, to show it is effective and practical. Even better, ask permission to have the client call the mentioned facility for more information;

- ✓ **Provide lists of resources and consultants** where the client can get help instituting the change.

IV. **Perceived self-efficacy.** The original Model design did not include this variable; the original research subjects, health screening, and immunizations, were considered simple behaviors requiring little skill aside from a strong intention to act within a short time span. However, as chronic conditions such as weight loss, smoking cessation, dental hygiene, and other life-altering conditions became more important in public health, the authors of the Model realized that behavioral changes required to influence those conditions would be more complicated. Chronic conditions, they stated, are "more difficult to surmount . . . [requiring] a good deal of confidence that one can . . . alter such lifestyles."[137] Therefore, this final step, perceived self-efficacy, was added to the Model design.

---

[137] Irwin M. Rosenstock, PhD, Victor J. Strecher, PhD, MPH, and Marshall H. Becker, PhD, MPH, "Social Learning Theory and the Health Belief Model," *Health Education Quarterly*, Summer 1988, 15(2): 175-183.

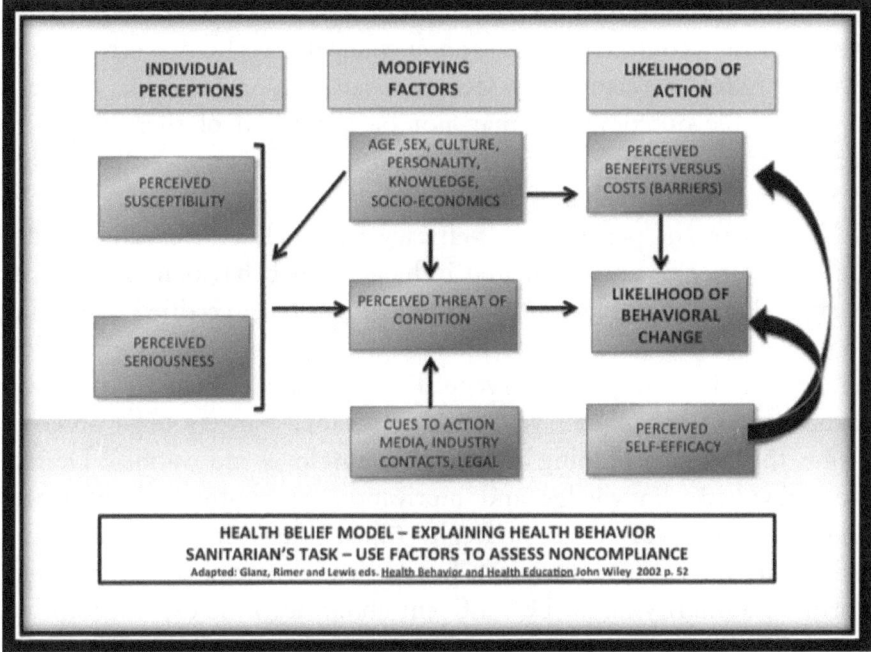

FIGURE 4: HEALTH BELIEF MODEL

Figure 4 is figure 3 adapted to include the factor of 'perceived self-efficacy'. It is implied in *barriers to action* and influences the individual's *likelihood of action* (third column). See Irwin M. Rosenstock, PhD, Victor J. Strecher, PhD, MPH and Marshall H. Becker, PhD, MPH, "Social Learning Theory and the Health Belief Model" *Health Education Quarterly (Summer, 1988: V. 15 (2) pp. 175-183)* for a discussion of the integration of social learning theory with the Model.

There are two components to perceived self-efficacy: efficacy and outcome expectations.[138] The two have a reciprocal influence: *outcome expectations*, the conviction that "a given behavior will lead to certain outcomes" must be strong enough to drive *efficacy expectations*, "the conviction that one can successfully execute the behavior required to produce [the recommended behavioral change]."[139] The two are distinct. On one hand, a person may feel confident that a behavior will lead to a desirable outcome but may not be persuaded of their ability to accomplish it. Or, in contrast, the person might feel sure of their ability to act but doubt the value of the outcome.

The factor of perceived self-efficacy was included to acknowledge the importance of environmental influences on behavioral change. For example, knowledgeable, motivated individuals (e.g., certified swimming pool operators or food service managers) may observe unsafe practices yet be lack the ability to intervene. During a site evaluation, they will acknowledge the problem yet speak of change barriers (e.g., absentee owner, the lack of a training budget, poor employee motivation). Despite the individual's knowledge and motivation, environmental influences slow the mastery of coping strategies (most often use of resources and skills to master coping strategies). In contrast, an inexperienced manager fearful of authority might be confident about outcome expectations but not about efficacy expectations.

Perceived self-efficacy is the most critical of all factors in the Model; inclusion of it acknowledges the importance of environmental motivators in behavioral change. A literature review suggests that this factor is the most statistically significant in predicting compliance with

---

[138] In this book, the term *outcome* and associated knowledge and skills concepts are associated with the abatement of a public health risk or concern. While sanitarian trainers often reference outcomes to the expectations of auditors, that should be a complementary step not an end in itself.

[139] Albert Bandura, *Social Learning Theory* (Englewood Cliffs, New Jersey: Prentice-Hall, 1977) p. 79

public health behavioral change.[140] [141] Bandura states that "perceived self-efficacy proved to be . . . a better predictor of behavior . . . than did past performance," and furthermore that "self-efficacy derived from partial *inactive* mastery during the course of treatment predicted performance on stressful tasks that the individuals had *never* done before"[142] (italics are mine).

Sanitarians need to consider both outcome and efficacy expectations during their site visit; an experienced, educated manager might have strong efficacy expectations, for example, but feel that the compliance outcome will be ineffective, counterproductive, or simply politically motivated. Furthermore, their strong efficacy expectations may be misleading if the specific nature of the task is misunderstood or is generalized. They may not prepare adequately for the task, leading to failure. Bandura stresses this point

> An aid to performance is a strong sense of self-efficacy to withstand failures coupled with some uncertainty (construed in terms of the challenge of the task rather than fundamental doubts about one's capabilities) to spur preparatory acquisition of knowledge and skills[143]

Ask this individual if he or she can train effectively, and the response might be, "I tell them what to do and then fire them if they don't do it! That's how I train." Of course, this "verbal persuasion" is far from effective and in no way constitutes effective training. The sanitarian must observe to determine how high perceived self-efficacy translates into

---

[140] Nancy K. Janz and Marshall H. Becker, "The Health Belief Model: A Decade Later," *Health Education Quarterly*, Spring 1984, 2(1): 1-47.

[141] James E. Maddux and Ronald W. Rogers, "Protection Motivation and Self-Efficacy: A Revised Theory of Fear Appeals and Attitude Change," *Journal of Experimental Social Psychology*, 1983, 19(5): 9.

[142] Albert Bandura, *Social Foundations of Thought & Action: A Social Cognitive Theory*, (Englewood Cliffs, New Jersey: Prentice-Hall, 1986).p. 261.

[143] Albert Bandura, "Self-efficacy Mechanism in Human Agency", *American Psychologist* v. 37 (2) 2/82 pp. 122-147 quote on page 123

reality. At times it might be necessary to advise a step backward to review and refresh needed knowledge and skills.

The importance of efficacy expectations "suggests that the effectiveness of personal interventions might be strengthened by explicit attention to ways of increasing people's conviction that they have the capability of performing actions that are needed to produce desired outcomes."[144] Thus, while it is vital for clients to understand *what* to do, *how* to do it, and *why* they should do it (the first stages of the Model), they fail most often because they believe they lack the *skills* for doing it. Given strong positive perceptions of all factors in the Model, clients still may fail due to a low perceived self-efficacy, a perception that they are unable to make the change. Even if a change is perceived as important (outcome expectations), it will not be attempted unless the individual believes in his or her ability to act (efficacy expectations).

To strengthen these convictions, it is vital for clients to accompany the sanitarian on the site evaluation. They can witness problems, and associated coping strategies, first hand and either practice or actively participate in corrections. The sanitarian can clarify and simplify the desired behaviors.

Not only does practice improve mastery of the specified coping strategy, but it also influences the potential for performing future, unspecified skills. (The tendency to comply will carry over to future site inspections and unspecified corrective actions.) This carries far more predictive power of behavior than an individual's vicarious observations of others or his or her stated intentions to act. However important the last two factors, they cannot take the place of having a chance to practice in a nonthreatening environment.

Self-efficacy also has a reciprocal influence on barriers to change: increased self-efficacy will make barriers seem less daunting[145] and vice versa. There also may be generalized effects of self-efficacy on self-esteem or self-confidence, possibly increasing motivation and intention to act

---

[144] Irwin M. Rosenstock, unpublished grant proposal.
[145] Albert Bandura, *Social Learning Theory* (Englewood Cliffs, New Jersey: Prentice-Hall, 1977) p. 79.

in other areas. Research has not yet been done in those areas, however.[146] Furthermore, increased motivation without *specific* skills training could be counterproductive and regressive if the individual performs a new behavior inadequately.

Both the person in charge (manager, supervisor) and employees must have a high level of perceived self-efficacy. During the inspection interview, the manager may express a high perceived self-efficacy for both skills and outcome. His or her perceived and *actual* control may be two entirely different things, however. If he or she is unable to train employees and effectively involve them in the change process, this control can never translate into reality.

The perceived ability to act is influenced by the client's cognitive and social environments, their attitudes and information about the recommended change, observations of others they respect or admire,[147] and their opportunity to practice and master the new behavior. Even if the client believes the change is important, they must also believe in their ability to act in the face of adverse conditions (barriers); otherwise, the proposed change will not be attempted. Social learning theory suggests that performing the action even once may prompt the client to try again until mastery is attained.[148] Self-efficacy will be greatly influenced by a credible model for the proposed behavior and adequate *sheltered* time to gain competency.

Here are some summary statements about what a strong level of perceived self-efficacy can accomplish:

- ✓ It determines whether or not people will even try to cope with difficult situations. Without high self-efficacy, the attempt might not even be made;

---

[146] Lyn Lawrence and Kenneth R. McLeroy, "Self-Efficacy and Health Education," *Journal of School Health,* October 1986, 56(8): 317-320.

[147] Sanitarians increase their credibility as models when they assume other respected social roles; e.g., teachers, community volunteers.

[148] Irwin M. Rosentock, PhD, Victor J. Strecher, PhD, MPH, and Marshall H. Becker, PhD, MPH, "Social Learning Theory and the Health Belief Model," *Health Education Quarterly*, Summer 1988, 15(2): 175-183.

- ✓ Once the initial attempt is made, high efficacy expectations determine how long that effort will last. It is important for the sanitarian, client and others to offer encouragement until mastery is achieved;

- ✓ Research shows that participant modeling is an important source of self-efficacy compared to the effects of vicarious observation of others. Sanitarians must provide time during site visits to allow modeling and practice;

- ✓ Vicarious observation of a wide range of different individuals, not just one model, serves to reinforce and encourage the participant to persist. "If people of widely differing characteristics can succeed, then observers have a reasonable basis for increasing their own sense of self-efficacy"[149].

A cautionary note goes with this lengthy discussion about Social Learning Theory. In the rush to compensate for prior neglect of environmental influences, a person's psychological readiness for change cannot be taken for granted. Rosenstock cautions that ". . . while the failure to measure self-efficacy in earlier research . . . was certainly an important omission, it is also an error to stake as much on self-efficacy as many . . . theories have . . . attempted".[150] Even with a comprehensive environmentally based intervention design, a noncompliant individual may still lack the motivation to change: the integration of the Model and Social Learning Theory are critical.

---

[149] Albert Bandura "Self-Efficacy: Toward a Unifying Theory of Behavioral Change" *Psychological Review* V. 84 (2) pp.191-215 bulleted points from pp. 193-197, quote on p. 197

[150] Irwin M. Rosenstock, Ph.D, Victor J. Strecher, Ph.D, MPH, and Marshall H. Becker Ph.D, MPH, "Social Learning Theory and the Health Belief Model" *Health Education Quarterly* V. 15(2) (Summer, 1988) pp. 175-183 more specifically p. 180

Suggestions for Sanitarians

Here are some ideas for sanitarians to consider: first, *outcome expectations* (confidence that a given behavior will resolve the problem) might be influenced in the following ways:

- ✓ *Maintain consistency throughout site evaluations, particularly in regard to high-risk concerns.* (Flexible compliance times are needed for concerns with low-risk public health impact where the expense may create an economic hardship.) This makes the inspection credible and predictable; clients will understand that compliance coping strategies have a scientific, not political, basis and will not change with different sanitarians and inspections.

    A predictable objection to this suggestion is that it restricts the individual sanitarian's professional discretion and creates a mechanical approach to site evaluations. There are many reasons why sanitarians must follow the same parameters for marking high-risk concerns; however, each sanitarian still faces unique and challenging tests of their communication and persuasive abilities.

- ✓ *Document the outcome's public health impacts* (positive and negative) to the client, through the use of newsletters, media, brochures and technical books. On the negative side, show how the failure to make corrections resulted in food-related illness, legal action, public relations problems or similar effects; on the positive side, show how the required changes are being instituted by other facilities or the industry as a whole;

- ✓ *Provide resources, references and recommended contacts* to help the supervisor choose the most effective and desirable compliance method. Include lists of approved materials and equipment, places to obtain products or hire consultants, compliance methods used by other facilities.

Outcome expectations are much easier for sanitarians to influence: fewer resources are needed; interventions can be conducted uninterrupted both at the site and in the office (mailings, telephone interviews, office conferences) and mechanisms such as mass media and networking are already in operation.

Efficacy expectations, however, are a different matter. Interventions must occur at the site, since activities involve employee education in core sanitation skills and risk monitoring. These activities are often foreign to sanitarians and site management; more resources must be expended to produce a positive result. Mechanisms in place for education and training, as has already been discussed, often were developed by using common but flawed designs that produce ineffective results.

Here are some general recommendations for sanitarians about *efficacy expectations*:

- ✓ *Model behaviors* [151] *and encourage practice,*[152] preferably during the site visit.[153] The net effect of modeling occurs whether or not it is consciously planned or enacted; employees observe and copy activities during the site visit. Sanitarians and site supervisors serve as models of 'correct' behavior (even if the behavior is far from correct!). For this reason, sanitarians must plan each site visit carefully. Equipment must be organized, calibrated

---

[151] Successful modeling also will influence the client's perception of source and message credibility. A sanitarian who adheres to the sanitation principles he or she enforces can expect closer attention from site personnel.

[152] Marshall Becker and Lois Maiman, "Strategies for Enhancing Patient Compliance," *Journal of Community Health*, Winter 1980, 6(2): 113-133. The authors discuss strategies such as "making [these] changes gradually over the course of several visits, taking the behaviors one at a time, reinforcing whatever compliance is achieved, and only then adding the next objectives . . ." (117-119). This, of course, will be useful only in cases of non-imminent risk.

[153] While precision is important for all activities, some environmental health services are not easily practiced (e.g., pumping a septic tank or installing a sewage disposal field). In these cases, verbally rehearse the activity and use audiovisual simulations as a substitute.

and in good working order prior to entering the facility site[154]. For example, at a swimming pool, have a chemical test kit with reagents and a flashlight; if the site is a food service, wash hands thoroughly, put on a head covering, and remove outdoor clothing before entering the kitchen.

- ✓ *Encourage skills* practice during the site visit.[155] While this is not always practical, especially during the busiest operating times, a certain amount of practice can occur along with observations of employee activities. Simulations can occur before and after the busiest operating hours. When a concern is noted and documented, use the time to model and practice the correct coping strategy.

- ✓ Maintain a positive or neutral learning process, **never** negative, even during the most hectic operating hours. Acknowledge positive aspects of the incorrect behavior (some portion of the behavior was correct) and reinforce them. Use positive examples during pre- and post-interviews, and use employees as models during training. While direct, hands-on practice is best, vicarious experience also may be effective if the models are respected staff members or if actual practice is impractical. Site personnel will use the positive reinforcement to build upon after the site evaluation is finished.

  During a site evaluation, observations and monitoring will reinforce positive behaviors and offer input for future training programs. In a swimming pool filter room, ask personnel to backwash the sand filter or use a chemical test kit to check sanitizer residuals. In a food service facility have site

---

[154] Employee observations will begin the minute the sanitarian drives onto the property.

[155] While precision is important for all activities, some environmental health services are not easily practiced (e.g., pumping a septic tank or installing a sewage disposal field). In these cases, verbally rehearse the activity and use audiovisual simulations as a substitute.

personnel assist in rearranging food storage, setting up the three-compartment sink, stocking the hand sink, or mopping the floor. While this is done under the guise of evaluating skills and knowledge, it gets personnel to adopt better habits.

It is inevitable that sanitarians will make mistakes during inspections and not know answers to some questions. Turn these instances into training experiences; acknowledge the mistake, find the correct answers, and use the moment to advantage. Discuss the error, ask for input on how the behavior should have occurred, and repeat it correctly. The staff will learn, and the sanitarian's credibility will improve.

- ✓ *Provide training during inspections.* Communicate to employees, through the supervisor,[156] what behavior is expected and how it is to be accomplished (see principles for training program design). Sanitarians should offer assistance with employee training by observing or co-teaching the program.

- ✓ *Use pre- and post-evaluation interviews to define and strengthen the link* between the unsafe behavior and the behavioral change, using handouts, newsletters and media releases.

- ✓ *Offer a compliance plan in installments,*[157] using a risk-assessment method, separating violations and compliance times by their relative risk. Explain to site personnel, that, while evaluative standards require full documentation and rapid compliance for high-risk concerns, there is discretion in the evaluation and abatement of low-risk concerns. A division of compliance times into phases will give management time for more effective employee training; compliance may be better as a result. Some

---

[156]

[157] Some sanitarians may object that this constitutes a rewriting of the law. However, clients always have been allowed to request time extensions on low-risk items; more frequent site visits could be used to verify higher-risk concerns. Codes often separate items into risk categories, so this is not a new idea.

clients will prefer to comply immediately with all requirements; realistic sub-goals will motivate others (especially inexperienced ones) toward better compliance. Sanitarians will need to keep records and do more short site visits to check on progress; the result may be better long-term compliance and better morale.[158]

- ✓ *Verbal persuasion.* This approach is common with supervisors who are both concerned about saving resources and convinced that skills acquisition is easy. However, while this method can prompt attention, it can be counterproductive if provided without coping strategies and training

- ✓ *Emphasize the benefits, **not** the costs of change.* While a credible evaluation must be balanced with a fair assessment of positive and negative aspects, be certain to emphasize the positive ones. Show how most sanitation improvements involve only effective training and little financial investment.

- ✓ *Revisit clients*, even after compliance seems assured, to reinforce good habits and offer assistance where relapse might occur. This probably should not be a formal evaluation, only a 'coffee break' type stop for the sanitarian to catch up with the client and answer questions.

Individuals change their behavior at different rates, influenced by different factors. Research suggests that there are stages of change, ranging over time periods up to six months (depending, of course, on the nature of change, and its relative severity and stress). Without reinforcement of incremental improvements, relapse is possible at any time during the time period. Use of the Model, and associated factors, is a dynamic, interactive process that must be revisited any number of times to assure consistent compliance with health concerns.[159]

---

[158] Albert Bandura, *Social Learning Theory*, (Englewood Cliffs, New Jersey: 1977) pp. 141 (realistic sub-goals), 162 (goal proximity).

[159] Martin Fishbein and Icek Ajzen, *Predicting and Changing Behavior: The Reasoned Action Approach* (New York: Psychology Press, 2010), pp. 353-357.

Despite these conditions, a strong perceived self-efficacy still has positive aspects,. Once a new behavior has been attempted and reinforced, and once self-efficacy has risen to mastery levels, the strategy will be attempted again until it is mastered.[160]

This will occur even *without any reinforcing presence* (sanitarian, management). The process can be shortened by the sanitarian's modeling the correct behavior and reinforcing an employee's attempt to practice it. With repetition and practice, these behaviors (e.g. setting up an ice water bath or the cleaning and sanitizing process at the pot and pan sink) will persist after the sanitarian has left and continue between routine inspections. Employees who master these skills become proactive in the facility, taking ownership of their work area and criticizing others who fail to meet these standards.

Perceived self-efficacy does not equate to self-confidence or self-esteem; increased self-efficacy does not translate to other specific behaviors or skills. It is logical, however, that mastery of one specific skill (e.g., preventing cross-contamination during food *preparation*) may result in a greater willingness to attempt a similar task (e.g., preventing cross-contamination in food *storage*). Without the proper training for the new task, however, this confidence could result in failure.

The enhanced version of the Health Belief Model, including the additional factor of perceived self-efficacy, is illustrated in figure 4. Self-efficacy has a reciprocal influence with the likelihood of action and perceived benefits (illustrated by arrows). As an individual becomes more confident of his or her ability to perform the change, both the benefits of the action and the likelihood of performing it increase. There also will be some generalized influence of high levels of perceived self-efficacy on socio-demographic factors.

---

[160] Irwin M. Rosenstock, Ph.D., Victor J. Strecher, Ph.D., MPH, and Marshall H. Becker Ph.D., MPH, "Social Learning Theory and the Health Belief Model" *Health Education Quarterly V. 15 (2)* (Summer, 1988) pp. 175-183

IMPLEMENTING CHANGES: INTRODUCTION TO INTERVENTION DESIGN

The preceding section discussed problems with the current approach to inspections and how the use of behavioral science concepts could better address noncompliance. The existing system concentrates on changing outcome behaviors, with no regard for the individual's attitudes, beliefs and motivations. The Model, and related behavioral science concepts, concentrate on explaining the role of attitudes, beliefs and motivations. That said, what is the best way to integrate the two approaches into the existing system?

Most sanitarians believe they are already accomplishing this; they discuss aspects of the Model (e.g., problem severity, problem susceptibility, cues to action, and general coping strategies) during their inspections, time permitting. They spend time talking to the client about these issues and offer opportunities for training and education.

There are two major problems, however: an incomplete understanding of behavioral science concepts influencing the client; and time limitations imposed by legal mandates and the evaluation report. While sanitarians genuinely attempt to address the client's concerns, these attempts are biased by psychodynamic assumptions about behavioral change. These limitations have already been discussed. Time limits usually dictates an emphasis on audit requirements, i.e. susceptibility, severity and coping strategies. This, in turn, leads to glossing over of concept distinctions and misunderstandings about the issues of causality.

As a result, the evaluation report is the focus of the site visit, not sanitation status. Clients anticipate the impending site visit,[161] discussing procedures and protocols with their staff and rehearsing possible responses to the site report. They have well-formed attitudes before

---

[161] Clients may know the sanitarian's schedule or that they are in the neighborhood.

the site visit takes place. Sanitarians must anticipate this fact with a well-designed intervention strategy.

An effective intervention must be based on the needs of specific target populations (client and/or employees). Since each cohort (e.g., ethnic restaurants and workers) will have different concerns, ad hoc research must be conducted during networking and/or site visits to better understand the population. Data must be gradually acquired during site inspections. Then the Health Belief Model and other behavioral science concepts can be applied to identify weak points preventing compliance.

The intervention must be designed based on two possible reasons for noncompliance: low self-efficacy (environmental) or a weak inclination to act (psychological). The existing enforcement-based strategy always assumes the latter, assuming that mitigating or modifying factors are inaccessible for analysis, except through the individual's self report. While this approach is easier to implement and affects more people, the effects will be varied and unpredictable. An intervention must be concerned with the motivational factors, "the primary beliefs that determine the behavior. [Otherwise] . . . such a message will often not be very effective and may even be counterproductive." [162]

The Health Belief Model and associated behavioral science concepts (e.g. social learning theory, reasoned action approach) are vital in addressing the issues surrounding a low perceived self-efficacy. As these concepts are integrated into the existing inspection intervention plan, education and consultation functions will gradually assume more importance and will be introduced earlier in the intervention strategy. Enforcement strategies, while still present and viable, will move to the background. This process will be gradual over time, as sanitarians must be trained to change inspection styles. Note that this will not be as radical as first assumed; many sanitarians already apply the Model, albeit not technically and not in name.

---

[162] Martin Fishbein and Icek Ajzen, *Predicting and Changing Behavior: The Reasoned Action Approach* (New York: Psychology Press, 2010), p. 339.

DESIGNING THE INTERVENTION

A properly designed intervention is a cyclical and dynamic process in which education, enforcement, and consultation complement and catalyze each other, influencing the client's intention to act. In reaching their intention to act, clients consider much more than the written inspection report (this may be why so many reports remain in desk drawers unread!) Sanitarians must consider that fact during their interventions for change.

An intervention is basically an attempt at problem solving, similar in structure and intent to any type of standard operating procedure, HACCP,[163] or other risk-control effort. A theoretical construct is described below, with the understanding that sanitarians will have to work with it section by section, accumulating data as they conduct site visits. Behavioral science principles should be kept close at hand, as they will influence the ultimate intervention design.

Intervention Step 1: Define the target behavior[164] and the target population.

This step seems obvious: the concerns, coping strategies (corrective actions), and target population are described in the inspection report. This is accurate in some high-risk cases, such as improper hand washing: the target behavior, coping strategy, and target population are all comingled. Other cases are not so clear, however; an observed outcome, even a high-risk concern such as unsafe food storage or cloudy swimming pool water may evolve from any number of unseen behaviors or populations. Low-risk concerns connected with infrastructure or equipment may have evolved naturally or out of neglect, with any number of target groups involved. Or, in other instances, the sanitarian may observe a fully developed situation with no activity: the causal behavior must be inferred.

---

[163] HACCP: hazard analysis and critical control points;—a risk assessment and control plan.

[164] Martin Fishbein and Icek Ajzen, *Predicting and Changing Behavior: The Reasoned Action Approach* (New York: Psychology Press, 2010), pp. 326-363.

Any number of people may be involved in the concern and the final coping strategy. There might be an absentee owner, a smaller subset of employees, or other government inspectors who are responsible (unintentionally, of course) for the infraction.[165] Those present at the inspection may be innocent bystanders. With little help from the client, who either has not seen the offense or wants to avoid a citation, the target population and target behavior (coping strategy) must be incorrectly identified. The sanitarian may need to ask some questions to determine exactly how the offending situation actually developed and how it should be resolved. Otherwise, the resulting intervention will be misdirected and quite possibly counterproductive. All of these factors indicate the need to tailor interventions toward the needs of individual populations and facilities, as well to revisit intervention design periodically when there are lapses in a facility's progress.

Step 2: Understand the client's state of mind.

After the target behavior is understood and the target population is defined, the prevailing mindset must be understood as well. This is a difficult task. In the past, it was made easier by the assumption that proper knowledge, skills, and resources are available but that the motivation is lacking. Enforcement was relied upon to "strengthen" motivation to act. In reality, however, the mindset could consist of any number of factors and is not so easily deduced.

Mindset is critical to the intervention design; it determines which factors receive the most emphasis. Sanitarians do not have the luxury of questionnaires and random samples to acquire needs assessment data: this information must be gathered incrementally during site visits. Little

---

[165] Other inspectors may have rules that contradict environmental health codes and inadvertently create sanitation concerns. Some plumbing codes, for instance, do not allow indirect waste disposal for food sinks, due to potential splash of nonpotable wastewater. This is in direct contradiction to health codes that require indirect waste disposal to protect against backup of nonpotable water into the sink. Restaurants may have problems installing screen doors with self-closing devices on emergency fire exits, due to local fire codes. This code conflict can result in pest problems.

accurate help can be expected from the client. Often, sanitarians must plunge ahead and work by trial and error.

While much can be learned through site observations, watching employees as they work, *pre- and post-inspection interviews are vital to learning the client's state of mind.*[166] In intervention design, "a crucial consideration . . . is whether people do or do not have the intention to engage in the behavior under consideration."[167] Interviews are a good place to discover this information. If the site visit is rushed, revisit at a later date.

Make interviews as compulsory as other audit and inspection standard procedures. Sanitarians and clients may both prefer to avoid them. Nevertheless, even just the offer of one is important; clients need to see the sanitarian as empathetic to their situation, interested in explaining and describing the inspection process. It shows respect for the client's "home",[168] gives them a chance to describe developments on-site[169], and focuses their attention on the public health problem, not on legal consequences. While sanitarians may be well versed in environmental topics and risk assessment, the perceptions and priorities of site personnel determine the success or failure of the intervention. The information is an essential component in an active intervention to change behaviors and improve public health status.[170]

---

[166] Some clients will not appreciate the interview, because it extends the site evaluation time; some sanitarians will be eager to leave some sites and clients behind. While the interviews would not be legal documents, they must be written so that the health agency has a database for future reference.

[167] This knowledge influences the design of the intervention, where attention is most needed, on attitudes or on self-efficacy. Martin Fishbein and Icek Ajzen, *Predicting and Changing Behavior: The Reasoned Action Approach* (New York: Psychology Press, 2010), p. 353.

[168] Many clients, especially ethnic populations, view their site as their "home" and the sanitarian as their "guest"

[169] Give the client a chance to discuss something positive that has developed since the last site visit, even if it is not related to sanitation. Sanitarians are often too busy to see these changes.

[170] F.M. Loewenberg, <u>Fundamentals of Social Intervention</u> (New York: Columbia University Press, 1977) p. 193.

These interviews are important to gather information, assess attitudes, answer questions, discuss industry and site developments, clarify future expectations, and allow the client to state their intentions to act in the future. Clients should also be asked about the coping strategy's practicality as well as about possible barriers that might keep them from performing the behavior properly.

Use an interview form (see the Appendix for examples) to note the client's attitudes, beliefs, state of mind, personal interests, intentions to act, and developments at the site. There will be situations in which use of the form or a formal interview is not practical; perhaps the site evaluation is outdoors, in inclement weather, or hurried. No matter the situation, it is essential to gauge the attitudes of site personnel. These processes, and the resulting information, have nearly as valuable an impact as identifying and acting upon public health hazards. The client begins to view the sanitarian as more than an enforcer, as someone interested in the future of the client and the facility. The sanitarian becomes more trustworthy and credible.

Even though the interview is not a formal portion of the inspection, it is a part of the facility's public record and is accessible through the freedom of information process. Therefore, never include privileged information such as recipes, economics, or client personal information (health, habits).

One important part of the interview process is asking clients to state their intention to perform the recommended behavior in the future. Fishbein and Ajzen state that "simply asking people when, where, and how they will carry out their intentions greatly increased the likelihood that they will do so."[171] A stated intention to act is strongly correlated to actual behavioral change, *modified by the client's perceived self-efficacy* (their volitional control over behavior; see the next paragraph). This request helps the client's memory (those with strong intentions to act simply forget to do it) and gives the impression of a contractual agreement.

This commitment must be specific and proximate, detailed and practical. For instance, the sanitarian may have noted a lack of consistent hand washing after personnel use the restroom. There might be a discussion

---

[171] Martin Fishbein and Icek Ajzen, *Predicting and Changing Behavior: The Reasoned Action Approach* (New York: Psychology Press, 2010), p. 358

during the post-inspection interview in which the client may be asked to validate a change: "I and my staff will immediately start washing hands after leaving the restroom, using soap and hot water and scrubbing for thirty seconds." This specific statement is important versus general assurances of improvement. This process must be done separately from the inspection process so the client will feel more comfortable discussing their plans and concerns. It must, however, be an official part of each site visit.

As information is gradually assembled through site visits and public health networking, it should be more apparent whether or not clients intend to act as recommended. If noncompliance persists, it is worthwhile to look at perceived self-efficacy. If the intention to act is weak, the intervention should not continue until resources are brought to bear on the client's attitudes and beliefs. A weak intention to act might indicate recalcitrance, but it also may indicate miscommunication about the nature of the problem, its immediacy, and its implications. At that point, the sanitarian needs to go back in the process and strengthen the areas where attitudes are weak or tentative.

USING THE MODEL DURING INTERVENTION DESIGN

In understanding and influencing the client's state of mind, the Model provides a good framework for this analysis. The appendix of this book provides some interview forms that might be used, after the initial needs assessment is complete, to assess possible points to intervene and influence the client's decision-making process. These forms suggest places where sanitarians can influence decision making. There is an intervention diagram, based on figures 3 and 4, to suggest areas where sanitarians might influence and speed compliance. A chart provides suggestions for actions in these areas. Finally there are two interview forms that can be used while talking with clients.

Does the individual believe the problem is immediate and severe? *The answer to this question may dictate the shape and scope of the developing intervention strategy.* If the person does not hold strong positive views, the intervention must start at that point, not proceed to influence behavioral change (although a series of steps might be addressed simultaneously).

As was mentioned earlier, sanitarians already spend considerable time on the first factors in the Model: problem severity, problem susceptibility, and cues to action. Often this effort consists of verbal persuasion (see below) and does not account for the client's state of mind; therefore, further time spent in these areas would likely be counterproductive.

Here are some additional approaches to consider when trying to understand and influence the client's beliefs:

- **Resources**. Keep a portfolio of fact sheets, pamphlets, and newsletters to use in persuading clients. Some sanitarians maintain plastic binders of information for each service program they administer. The sanitarian thus becomes a credible and trustworthy source of information; the client finds it more difficult to dismiss this source.

- **Patience.** Downplay enforcement potential until the client's attitudes are clearly developed or violations require an overt presence (this is more realistic where multiple site visits are expected or concerns are low-risk). This practice suggests the sanitarian's interest in the facility while retaining enforcement as a viable future option

- **Divide up larger tasks** to simplify and clarify requirements. For example, low-risk concerns such as structural or equipment damage might be scheduled in phases, with more frequent revisits as needed. Clients will be less likely to misunderstand and more likely to attempt corrections.[172]

- **Extend influence** into the client's community (see Model factor "Age, Sex, Culture, Personality, Knowledge, Socioeconomics") by . . .

    - *Networking,* with both industry and other health professionals, to disseminate and explain new rules communitywide as well as to provide external cues to influence clients. Use the system already established for community disaster response on a reduced scale to discuss this information. Have a database of environmental health topics available to the public by telephone or computer. Such a network will also help to better delineate and explain the different public health areas of expertise.

    - After the network is in place, if physicians, nurses, or industry representatives are asked a question related to environmental health, they will either (a) be able to reflect the sanitarian's message on the subject; (b) provide the client with printed materials conveying that message; or, if unsure of the message, make a referral to the environmental health offices.

    - *Providing publicity* for positive public health trends in the community or at sites; hold a media event to celebrate a

---

[172] Albert Bandura, *Social Learning Theory,* (Englewood Cliffs, New Jersey: Prentice-Hall, 1977) pp. 83-84.

site's improvements. If a facility shows positive trends or new sanitation ideas, ask if these can be recommended to others.

- *Working with mass media.* Public service announcements provide information but also serve as external cues to action. *Designate* media representatives within the health agency for consultations and feedback, as well as regular press releases. Distribute pamphlets, newsletters, and publicity about the health agency to the community through libraries, schools, and other community outlets. These campaigns reinforce the sanitarian's credibility as well as influence the client's trusted professional contacts in the community.

- *Making appearances at community events.* Sanitarians should develop a *community presence* by appearing at non-work-related events (seminars, educational programs, fairs, exhibits, school vocational days). In this way, sanitarians appear in roles other than an enforcement officer.

- *Encouraging school public health programs* on subjects such as hygiene, disease prevention, or general environmental health concerns so children take home sanitation concepts to their parents (clients).

• **Promote consistency**, in both positive and negative (legal) reinforcement, so clients will know what to expect to result from their behavior. For instance, the resolution of low or variable-risk concerns might vary with the situation and client; other high-risk items, however, should receive the same treatment by all sanitarians, regardless of site or client. Clients should be aware of this so they can 'accurately assess existing conditions of reinforcement (i.e. legal action) and avoid being 'lead . . . astray by erroneous expectations'.[173] Inconsistent reinforcement,

---

[173] Albert Bandura, *Social Learning Theory*, (Englewood Cliffs, New Jersey: Prentice-Hall, 1977) p. 167.

especially of high risk sanitation concerns, can delay compliance and create worse public health concerns.

- **Be persuasive.** Sanitarians must understand each citation and public health reasons for them. It is neither persuasive nor credible to give a reason such as 'it's the law'. If there is uncertainty about a concern or coping strategy, say so and return with the correct information. Hold regular staff meetings so that supervisors and sanitarians agree on the message the client will receive.

- **Sanitarians must be well versed in legal protocols** (injunction, warrant, testimony) so that legal actions, when needed, proceed efficaciously. Knowledge of legal protocols, especially the specialized concerns of environmental health, protects against the loss of legal actions in court. Legal action, when needed, should be consistently applied and effective. Such action tells the community what to expect in cases of persistent noncompliance.

- **Pursue professional education and training.** Review industry standards for equipment and processes so coping strategies are understood. Provide training programs to emphasize the public health impact of the various noncompliant behaviors.

- **Listen to the community.** Pay regular visits to local government outlets; discuss community concerns with representatives there. Subscribe to the community newspaper or, better, read it at the local library (libraries themselves are an informal information mill).

MAKING A PERSUASIVE ARGUMENT FOR CHANGE

In order to influence the client's beliefs and attitudes and reinforce the weaker points of the Model, sanitarians need to know how to communicate effectively and tailor a persuasive argument for change. At first, the concept of communication campaigns might not seem applicable to the sanitarian's work; under a specialized bureaucracy, it is typically a health education function. It also appears to be a abstract, cookie-cutter type function generalized across all types of public health messages. This misconception is due, in part, to a misunderstanding, both of the nature of site evaluations as well as the true nature of the sanitarian's function. Once it is accepted that site evaluations extend beyond a single stop, through to the attainment of acceptable sanitation status, the sanitarian's work then can be viewed as a communication campaign. The start of that campaign is an assessment function (site evaluation) followed by messages and education programs to inform, and persuade the client to change behaviors. The information and skills needed by site personnel are also delivered in different venues-on-site, in education programs, and within public health networks.

Therefore, the components typically reserved for public relations and media experts can be applied to the sanitarian's work. Unfortunately, due to misconceptions described earlier, sanitarians often are not exposed to these concepts and skills. First there is the essential skill of relating a concept's public health importance. Can all clients understand to a level adequate to change behaviors, why wiping cloths must be stored in a sanitizing solution, why a septic tank outlet pipe must have a vented elbow, or why a swimming pool skimmer basket must have a weir or double basket installed? The rationale used to persuade must be more than stating, "it's the law" or "reasonable people should be persuaded". If readers have followed the arguments thus far, those statements no longer are persuasive.

The credibility of the communication campaign will influence the client's attitude and subsequent intention to act. It is better to downplay the legal citation of the concern until a persuasive rationale can be found for citing it. In fact, it is sometimes best not to cite the concern at all if it cannot be persuasively communicated. During a stressful inspection, it makes sense to use all communication tools available. Otherwise, one ineffective message will discredit the entire source.

Source of Message

The client's receipt of the message will be influenced by his or her view of the sanitarian and any other contacts with the public health agency and its representatives. These might include other sanitarians, doctors, nurses, nutritionists, and health educators. There might be contacts with the governing body. So, while the sanitarian may deliver the message, the client may perceive the actual source as any number of other people or groups.

The client must see the sanitarian as credible, trustworthy, and *similar* to himself or herself.[174] McGuire states that, while research results are not conclusive on the subject, "peer sources . . . prove surprisingly effective . . . [when] pitted against experts."[175] Credible professionals include physicians, scientists, educators, and bankers. The sanitarian's message will have considerably more influence if doctors, nurses, and teachers also deliver it; hence the importance of public health networking. A sanitarian will also be more persuasive if he or she is also a doctor (rare but possible) or an educator (more likely, such as a teacher of food safety).

The sanitarian can empathize with clients by learning more about their life interests and culture outside of the their job. Learning a few words of another language and understanding aspects of a person's culture show respect and interest.

---

[174] A highly credible source might be counterproductive if clients do not believe it is also emphatetic. It is important for sanitarians to use all opportunities to escape their enforcement persona (community involvement, interviews during inspections, non-work-related conversation). Martin Fishbein and Icek Ajzen, *Predicting and Changing Behavior: The Reasoned Action Approach* (New York: Psychology Press, 2010), p. 339.

[175] William McGuire, "Theoretical Foundations of Campaigns", in Ronald E. Rice and William J. Paisely, eds., *Public Communication Campaigns* (Beverly Hills, London: Sage, 1981) p. 46.

The message should clearly link the concern, the coping strategy, and the sanitarian's intent to push for behavioral change. While this may increase resistance to the message, it will be "more likely to enhance persuasive impact . . . [by] . . . clarifying the message."[176] While audit standards require a statement of legal consequences for noncompliance, this may not be the same thing in the client's mind, especially if the sanitarian is not persuasive beyond that statement.

The message should be positive (as much as possible) and should be delivered as quickly as possible. Of course, accomplishing these things is a balancing act for the sanitarian. Concerns and their legal consequences cannot be omitted or glossed over, for fear of underemphasizing their importance. Audit evaluators do not like inclusion of positive comments for fear that they will be misunderstood. Still, it is always possible to comment on positive trends when they are observed; while each problem or concern in the report must be discussed, it is possible to review some areas quickly if the client is clearly familiar with them.

Communicating the message

If clients respect the message source as credible and trustworthy, they may pay better attention to the message. Beyond that point, however, there is no guarantee of a change in behavior. There is a conditional probability of success at different stages of message delivery: exposure, attention, liking, comprehension, skill acquisition, attitude change, information retention, information retrieval, and behavioral change. So even if a client sits with the sanitarian and listens to the report, there are many more hurdles before any behavioral change can result.

At this point in the process, an evaluation report is delivered to the client about the observed concerns and required changes. This report must be persuasive. Psychodynamic theory would suggest that this does not matter a great deal, that the message is common sense and should be accepted by reasonable people. At this point in the book, however, that theory has been dismantled. The client will have his or her own set

---

[176] William McGuire, "Theoretical Foundations of Campaigns," in Ronald E. Rice and William J. Paisely, eds., *Public Communication Campaigns* (Beverly Hills, London: Sage, 1981), p. 47.

of information, attitudes, and beliefs, creating cognitive dissonance and intellectual static, easily distorting the meaning of the report.

So, communications must be done with great care if the groundwork is to be laid for behavioral change. It is a difficult and nerve-racking business, communication. It was Mark Twain who said, "there are two kinds of speakers in the world: those that are nervous and those that are liars." There are many texts about the mechanics of public speaking and communication principles. Here are a few general pointers on how to prepare:

- *Remember the KISS principle.* Attributed to New York State Senator Chauncey Depew, and more recently Clarence Leonard Johnson[177], that principle says, "Keep it simple, stupid." Tell them what you're going to say, say it, and tell them what you just said. Most people do not recall more than 10 percent of what is said during a presentation: be sure it is the important 10 percent!

- *Speak to a select audience.* Be certain the message is delivered to the people who will use the behavior or skill being discussed. That may be as difficult as determining the client's mindset. On-site, the problem will be getting the message out to the employees who need to use the information. Typically, the site report will be discussed with only a few select individuals, leaving many others uninformed. In an education program, the opposite is true. Management typically will invite too many people to attend, incorrectly believing that participants not directly involved will use the information sometime in the future. This approach makes employees hate training, however; on that day, training will seem boring and dull, and by the time the material is useful, they will have forgotten what they heard and what is expected of them.

- *Ask for help.* Inexperienced clients (or sanitarians) training for the first time should ask someone to give support and offer

---

[177] Ben R. Rich, *Clarence Leonard (Kelly) Johnson: 1910-1990 A Memoir* (Washington, DC: National Academies Press, 1995) p. 13

suggestions for the next time. Client trainers might have an experienced employee assist with the training; sanitarians might conduct initial site evaluations with the trainer or another sanitarian. Occasional team teaching and team inspections also can be helpful.

- *Use audiovisual materials* to reinforce the program's main points. This reinforces important materials and also organizes the program. While humor and animation are useful tools to keep the audience interested, the main focus must always be the program information.

- *Apply* the principles of communication campaigns discussed elsewhere in this book.

- *Learn the principles of public speaking and adult learning.* See the section below on adult learning. To gain practice and expertise, sanitarians need to make presentations to community groups.

How should the message be structured and delivered? The answer to this question will apply equally well to formal education efforts and site evaluations. We deal first with site evaluations, and later we move to consider education programs.

Suggestions for Sanitarians

Here are some ideas for sanitarians to consider when designing media and communication campaigns.

- *Repeat* the message on different occasions, with different media (fact sheets, newsletters, videos, demonstrations); check with the client to be sure the message, and associated behavior, have been understood (i.e., "How are you progressing with problem X? That's a tough one, isn't it? Have you run into obstacles you'd like to discuss? Would you like to review it?"). If this is done properly, it shows empathy for a client having difficulty with a task. Provide the same information on the report, on fact sheets, or in newsletters. Be certain the client is on applicable mailing lists. Environmental health issues are often complicated—repeating the message aids the client in retention and makes the message's importance clear.

- *Verbal and written reminders* have been shown to strengthen a person's intention to act. Fishbein and Ajzen note that when people are asked why they 'failed to act on their intentions, (they) often mention that they simply forgot or that it slipped their mind(s)'[178] One study shows that postcard reminders were more effective 'cues to action' than no reminder at all[179]; another study concludes that 'the highest rate of vaccination occurred among recipients of the Health-Belief-Model postcard'[180]

- *Be positive.* Always include positive remarks about improvements observed during the site visit. If audit rules do not allow positive comments, mention them to the client during the inspection. If nothing positive is apparent, ask the client if there is anything new since the last site visit. No matter how negative the report may be, make it a point to find at least one positive comment about the facility, management, or employees;

- *Be brief.* See the KISS note above, as well as the note about rapid ("brief") speaking; this also applies to interviews. Audit standards require a comprehensive, accurate report with thorough explanations. However, if the client has observed a concern and

---

[178] Martin Fishbein and Icek Ajzen, *Predicting and Changing Behavior: The Reasoned Action Approach* (New York: Psychology Press, 2010), p. 358

[179] N. K. Janz and M. H. Becker, "The Health Belief Model: A Decade Later," in *Health Education Quarterly*, Spring 1984, 11(1): 1-47. The latter article cites a study in which postcard reminders were more effective "cues to action" than no reminder at all (p. 17).

[180] Eric B. Larson, James Bergman, Fred Heidrich, Barbara L. Alvin and Ronald Schneeweiss, 'Do Postcard Reminders Improve Influenza Vaccination Compliance?: A Prospective Trial of Different Postcard Cues' *Medical Care* V. 20 (6) (June, 1982) pp. 639-648 quote in abstract

demonstrates comprehension, do not belabor the point; move on to the next item.

- *Anticipate client objections.* Clients will anticipate barriers standing in the way of compliance; they also may have objections of their own. Try to anticipate these and raise them during the interview process; if in doubt, ask the client what barriers they anticipate (use the form in the Appendix to note these concerns). Discuss barriers to change openly and offer help in dealing with them.[181]

Designing Education Efforts

In any program design, for sanitarians or clients, there are two training objectives: knowledge and use of public health risk concepts (concepts mastery and attitude change); and the integration and mastery of behavioral science skills (aptitude change). Due to resource limits and evaluation difficulties, the temptation is to emphasize the former objective: this results in distorted evaluation results.

Education and communication processes have only just begun when participants take their seats in the classroom or when they sit down to review the inspection report. The process of changing behaviors is much more complicated than a classroom lecture, certainly more so than is implied by the style adopted by most educators. Incorrect assumptions about the nature of adult learning lead educators (and sanitarians) to assume that "increasing people's knowledge . . . [is] a goal which is worthy of attainment in itself . . ." [182] Psychodynamic theory assumes that, given this information, reasonable people will change their attitude

---

[181] William McGuire, "Theoretical Foundations of Campaigns," in Ronald E. Rice and William J. Paisely, eds., *Public Communication Campaigns* (Beverly Hills, London: Sage, 1981), p. 49 "It is wise to mention rather than ignore possible counterarguments against one's position . . ."

[182] T. E. Dielman, Sharon L. Leech, Sharon L. Marshall, H. Becker et al., "Dimensions of Children's Health Beliefs," *Health Education Quarterly*, Fall 1980, 7(3): 219-238.

and develop an intention to act. This, of course, is faulty thinking, made even more difficult by a faulty intervention design.

In addition to the focus on lecturing, however, there is the mistake of not stating behavioral objectives. For some reason, educators assume that stating educational goals will offend program participants, that the goals should somehow be obvious. While children can be instructed by rote memorization with long-term objectives, adults search for relevancy and applications for what they learn. In a vocational setting, with high-risk public health stakes, uncertainty wastes resources and could create a disaster. Sanitarians should not be content with this, and neither should educators. One would hardly call a program efficacious if final applications of knowledge were not measured or were left to chance.

Program planners often claim that the information is provided, abstractly, and there is no behavioral application anticipated. The information is useful or entertaining and participants will use it later. However, since the program objectives are not defined, participants will either use the information spuriously and nonproductively or not all. Resources and time will be lost, as well as enthusiasm for future training programs.

The planning and administration of education efforts is complicated. McGuire describes a "persuasion matrix" with five input variables and twelve dependent output variables.[183] There is a complicated process, after information is received, before it can be applied to behavioral change. The *empty vessel fallacy* (e.g., participants will accept information without condition) and the *attenuated effects fallacy* (e.g. the likelihood that a communication campaign or program will lead to behavioral change is not automatic but a conditional probability) warn against optimistic expectations from education programs.

If one hundred people attend an education program, they will be exposed to the program's information. Before they decide to act as recommended, however, they must *listen* to the message, be *interested* in it, *understand* it, agree it is *worthwhile* (attitude change), feel *capable* of acting on it (self-efficacy), and *remember* it long enough to act on it.

---

[183] William McGuire, "Theoretical Foundations of Campaigns," in Ronald E. Rice and William J. Paisely, eds., *Public Communication Campaigns* (Beverly Hills, London: Sage, 1981), pp. 41-70

David Mikkola, R.S., M.P.H.

It is optimistic to believe that all participants who initially hear the message will complete *all* of the required steps for behavioral change. Yet most health agencies assume exactly that, citing program attendance as a *direct* measure of program effectiveness. While participation is a worthy objective, it is only one of many perquisite steps. Unless administrators need an inexpensive, easy measure of program effectiveness or are simply not interested in the impact on behavioral change (both rather cynical conclusions), this is a strange measure. Evaluators of food service management certification programs, for example, attempt to justify those programs by suggesting a link between examination scores and improved sanitation status at the facility. When research appears to demonstrate success, it was done soon after the program ended, when there likely will be coincidental improvements due to a heightened motivation and positive attitude. On the whole, however, any improvements are short-lived. Sanitarians see this fallacy first hand when a certified manager does not recognize high-risk sanitation concerns or is unable to train employees effectively.

There's small wonder that these studies rarely show a significant improvement in sanitation status! In reality, a well-instructed program might have an examination pass rate of 80 percent; i.e., 100 x 80, or eighty participants, will provide enough correct answers to pass the examination. Depending on the examination, a passing rate might mask a loss of 20 to 25 percent of the information, perhaps the same information needed to improve status on-site.[184] In a food service operation, for instance, an individual might successfully pass an examination without remembering vital information such as safe food temperatures. When an educational program cannot offer skills training, it is even more vital that program graduates retain critical information linked to the success of their facility.

---

[184] The author taught food safety certification for twenty-five years; it was not unusual to see participants pass an exam yet miss critical food safety questions such as safe food temperatures. Statistically, this lack of information accounts for a majority of foodborne illness cases.

For purposes of this discussion, assume that eighty participants who pass the examination remember *all* information correctly[185]. Now, in addition to answering an examination question accurately, did they also understand the information,[186] feel it was useful, *and* feel capable of acting upon it? Will they remember it long enough to use it effectively outside the program, at their facility? It is reasonable to assume that of the original one hundred participants, perhaps ten to fifteen will finally attempt to change behaviors as recommended. And, since there will not be a model of the behavior to use as guidance, or any reinforcement from the sanitarian, the result might be incorrect and counterproductive. This may be one reason why health agencies require certified managers to become recertified. As an example of reasonable program expectations, McGuire cites one program's goal of between 2 and 10 percent success.[187]

With all of these disadvantages limiting program effectiveness, it becomes even more important to design the program as carefully and completely as possible. Here are some general observations (and recommendations for their use, both during site evaluations and during education programs); note that most of them also are important for increasing client self-efficacy (next section):

- **Describe the desired result.** Link knowledge in the classroom with the desired behavioral change; provide a clear step-by-step model of *what* to do and *how* to do it. It is critical that both "what" and "how" are included in the behavioral change and the practice model.

---

[185] An optimistic assumption. Exam scores show that most graduates correctly answer seventy-five to eighty-five percent of the questions. This might include two-thirds of critical sanitation concerns, if retained long enough to be useful.

[186] Remembering the information long enough to write it down does not mean it was understood.

[187] William McGuire, "Theoretical Foundations of Campaigns", in Ronald E. Rice and Paisely, eds., *Public Communication Campaigns* (Beverly Hills, London: Sage, 1981), p. 51.

- **Show relevancy.** Never invite employees to be trained because they *might* use the information someday. Be clear from the start how the information will be used. Adults are eager to learn if they know they have a use for the knowledge or skill. "Learning is a means to an end, not an end in itself."[188]

- **Define objectives.** Do not leave that task to the participants, but clearly define the end goal for the program or instruction. "Adults who are motivated to seek out a learning experience do so primarily . . . because they have a use for the knowledge . . . learning is a means to an end, not an end in itself."[189] Bandura notes that "people do not learn much from repeated paired experiences unless they recognize that events are correlated.", i.e. clearly linked[190].

- **Clarify expectations.** Adult learners "prefer single-concept, single-theory courses that focus heavily on the application of the concept to relevant problems. This tendency increases with age."[191]

- **Demonstrate.** Use a credible model to demonstrate the new behavior just described, a respected source who will reassure the others that the behavior can be done properly and will be an effective solution. The manager or key employees are good examples (**not** the sanitarian).

- **Practice.** Hold the education session in a place where all participants can practice the new behavior. Insist on this even

---

[188] Ron Zemke and Susan Zemke "30 Things We Know for Sure About Adult Learning" *Training* 7/88 pp. 57-61 quote on p. 58

[189] Ron Zemke and Susan Zemke, "30 Things We Know for Sure About Adult Learning" *Training* 7/88 pp. 57-61, quote on p. 58

[190] Albert Bandura, *Social Learning Theory*, (Englewood Cliffs, New Jersey: Prentice-Hall, Inc. 1977) pp.165.

[191] Ron Zemke and Susan Zemke "30 Things We Know for Sure About Adult Learning" *Training* 7/88 pp. 57-61 quote on pg. 58

if someone claims to know the behavior well. It is important that employees have a chance to make mistakes in a neutral, nonthreatening environment, to gain mastery of it before applying it in a real-life situation. If the behavior is complicated, divide it up into small, incremental steps.

- **Provide support.** There are times when training programs cannot be held at times or places where practice is practical. The enrollment may be too large, the space too small, the time inadequate, or the skill too complicated to allow it. Consider the possibility of rescheduling or redesigning the program. At the very least, simulate or rehearse the new behavior. Otherwise, provide a strong support system to assist employees on-site. Arrange for more frequent site visits to reinforce their efforts; provide checklists, worksheets, or other written reminders in case people forget what to do. Networking can be helpful in this regard, as reminders may already be circulating in the community.

Modeling and practice are extremely important training components. They have been abandoned, however, along with organized educational training efforts, using the real but incidental barrier of increased short-term resource costs. Supervisors anxious about their ability to educate employees create shortcuts to get around their principles. Shortcuts include a lecture format (classroom learning), vicarious experience, self-directed video learning modules, shadowing other employees, emotional arousal (fear), and verbal persuasion. Most have been discussed to some extent in previous sections. While short term costs are real enough, long term benefits (fewer call backs for repeated training, consistent behavioral change) are also real. Nothing takes the place of hands on learning experiences.

The problem with classroom lecture formats, and its correlation with behavioral change, has been discussed: lectures do not include hands on skills training. Learning through observations ('shadowing') does not give the employee direct hands-on experience learning the new skill. The effects of verbal persuasion and emotional arousal may motivate for a short time, but the effects decay quickly when the source of the motivation is no longer present. In sum, while these ideas may be useful in increasing levels of self-efficacy, gains are short-lived compared to those from direct experience performing the behavior.[192] Improvements in self-efficacy "are likely to be weak and short-lived . . . [however] . . . in order to change, people need corrective learning experience." (i.e. trying the skill for themselves and getting feedback on their progress.)

---

[192] Albert Bandura, *Social Learning Theory* (Englewood Cliffs, New Jersey: Prentice-Hall, Inc. 1977) pp. 78-85.

ACTUAL VERSUS PERCEIVED CONTROL

At this point in the intervention, we assume the client's attitude and intention to act are strong, education efforts have progressed well and things are on track for a change in behavior. The Health Belief Model has been integrated into the site evaluation process and the sanitarian is satisfied that the person in charge has a high level of perceived self-efficacy. The question now is whether or not this information translates into action. At this stage, the sanitarian needs to evaluate the information obtained about the client's mindset, whether or not it is reflected in reality.

Clients may be overly positive during their site inspection interviews, hoping to avoid any further problems and to end the inspection quickly. Now, it is important to evaluate the true situation by observing the client's control over employees and the facility in general. If the client indicated a strong perceived self-efficacy in an interview (i.e., they believe they are capable of performing the behavior), how strong is their *actual* control over employees and the facility? Is the client on-site full time, or must they work at other jobs or go to other sites? Is there an absentee owner who approves all actions and must be consulted? How much control does the client have to see that the recommended behavior occurs consistently and correctly? In other words, the client may have all the necessary requisites for compliance save one: effective control over employees or the facility. This conclusion will change the nature of the intervention.

In many cases, *actual* control will be different than what was perceived (by the sanitarian or the client). In other cases, there will be problems in both areas. In that case, the sanitarian will need to change roles from evaluator to educator and consultant. Models of correct behavior will be needed, and practice sessions should be provided until the client and employees have raised their skill levels and can proceed independently.

Earlier, recommendations were offered for strengthening the client's self-efficacy. While there is overlap to this phase, the following are recommendations for following up on those earlier efforts. Here are some recommendations for improving and strengthening client control:

Evaluating Intervention Efforts

Hopefully at this stage, the client has followed the phases of the Health Belief Model and now has started some type of compliance program. The sanitarian must evaluate that effort on an ongoing basis to be sure the progress continues.

- **Maintain organized notes** on the progress of the various clients and facilities, so that there is continuity between sanitarians.

- **Revisit clients** periodically to be sure progress is ongoing, perhaps halfway between formal site visits, to answer questions and assess the facility's progress. Be certain the client does not view this as a formal inspection.

- **Work to develop public health networks at all stages of intervention.** The concept of networking has been referenced at other points in this book (see "**Using the Model During Intervention Design**"). Networking is much more than a talking point; it is a valuable supplemental resource at all stages of the Health Belief Model. Other public health professionals regularly deliver environmental health information to their clients; coordinating this activity would assure its accuracy as well as provide a valuable support system for the sanitarian. At present, many different professional groups (public health professionals, police, firefighters, local government officials, media representatives, librarians, industry groups, and school system employees) deliver public health information to their clients, some of it inaccurate, some incomplete. The committee structure is already in place for handling community emergencies such as epidemics or terrorist alerts; the same system could be used, with less frequency and priority, to coordinate the release of public health information.

If the health agency has a trained public health media representative, the message could be disseminated through newspapers, press releases, media interviews, public seminars, and literature. This practice would show the sanitarian to be a respected and credible community resource but also to be someone acting outside of their enforcement persona. As an additional cue to success, this network might also include examples of facilities that regularly comply with the law; some health agencies have awards and recognition for facilities with a lower risk status.

VALIDITY QUESTIONS

Since the Model was designed to address *personal* preventative health behaviors, there will be some loss of predictive power in applying it to public *venues* such as a restaurant, swimming pool, or school. There also will be different attitudes and mindsets from site personnel with different levels of involvement and authority. (Some personnel may even carry more authority, albeit unofficially, than the formal supervisor or manager.) While the degree of variation must be confirmed by research, the author's experience suggests that this is a minor concern: most site personnel reject the point, stating they still use the environmental service personally (eat food, swim in a pool) and therefore have an obligation to the community to comply. It also is possible that these different attitudes, mindsets, and self-efficacy levels fall into environmental modifying factors, just as the community impacts personal habits. The correlation loss will vary from site to site and will need to be considered during each intervention.

Many health educators have criticized any attempt to carry over theories from personal preventative health behaviors to environmental health. An answer to this objection has already been cited earlier in this book. The Health Belief Model's authors made amendments to include the influences of environmental factors, adding the factor of perceived self-efficacy. There are numerous examples of health education books applying health behavior research to environmental health concerns such as food safety, air pollution mitigation, hazardous waste disposal, and the like.[193] A recent effort by Frank Yiannis runs parallel to the efforts in this book to integrate behavioral science concepts with environmental health. To quote from the book description

---

[193] Richard B. Dwore and Joseph Matarazzo, "The Behavioral Sciences and Health Education: Disciplines with a Compatible Interest?" *Health Education*, May/June 1981, pp. 4-7.

> In fact, simply put, food safety equals behavior . . . Thus, to improve food safety, we need to better integrate food science with behavioral science and use a systems-based approach to managing food safety risk.[194]

The integration of behavioral science, health education and environmental health is not just an academic exercise but a synthesis actively pursued.

Finally, sanitarians may dismiss this book as spurious and unrealistic in the real world. They may claim they are already utilizing a holistic approach, as much as audit standards allow. Any more changes would be considered to be impossible to sustain financially and to be unnecessary. It is difficult to abandon the tempting notion of client as recalcitrant, especially during a stressful site evaluation. However, sanitarians (including the author and others) regularly stretch audit standards to include Model factors and improve compliance. While sanitarians on the whole do an admirable job balancing the political and social pressures of their job, the profession can be improved by addressing the concerns in this book. Reliance on enforcement has not addressed noncompliance issues; changes are needed. Those changes can easily be addressed within the existing system, while still upholding the profession's integrity.

---

[194] Frank Yiannis, *Food Safety Culture: Creating a Behavior-based Food Safety Management System* (New York: Springer Publications 2009) Cited as an example of behavioral science applications to environmental health. Book description quoted from Amazon.com web site.

SUMMARIZING THE NEED FOR CHANGE

Many potential applications have been discussed above; nevertheless, there is a matter of how quickly and extensively to begin implementation. The sanitarian's work is influenced, and often driven, by numerous social, political, and economic factors, deeply entrenched in an enforcement persona. Progress and change are frustrated by the inconsistency of coworkers and administrators, not to mention confrontations with clients. There is hardly time in a site visit to complete existing evaluative requirements, let alone add to that the activities described in this book. These changes seem extensive, expensive, time-consuming, and largely impractical.

In spite of these drawbacks, change may be more seamless and natural than first appears. The sanitarian's original academic training was grounded in a holistic application of enforcement, engineering, and education; changes can occur rapidly once administrators provide impetus and evaluators provide flexibility. Sanitarians, including the author, already apply these concepts independently within the current enforcement-based envelope.

Sanitarians would not be working alone in this effort: other public health professionals would work within networks to disseminate and clarify public health information. Public health change has synergy; as individuals successfully change personal health behaviors, this influences attitudes about possibly changing others. Active networks, along with consistency and changes in evaluative standards, would encourage individual sanitarians to adopt this holistic perspective.

Sanitarians would not be expected to shoulder the entire burden of change; networking, both intra- and inter-agency venues, must play an assertive and significant role. In addition, the intent of this book is not to redefine the inspection process, but only to suggest alternative means to evaluate and explain noncompliance. There is only so much change that can be effected during a site evaluation; only so much information can be distributed and absorbed. Sanitarians are only one part of the equation.

The theories used in this discussion are included to give a solid scientific foundation to proposals that otherwise might be misconstrued as ivory-tower, wishful thinking. While the Health Belief Model was used, there are many similar models, all of which intermix the influences of psychological and environmental influences on behavioral change. The important point is to explore all available explanations of noncompliance. These theories are provided to show that this discussion is neither new nor unrealistic. *The point is not to develop amateur behavioral scientists* but rather to expand the capacity to intervene with clients.

With all of these caveats in mind, the next step is to implement change.

STEPS TO IMPLEMENTATION

It is now time to discuss the design and implementation of the new system. Most of the system and the evaluation process will look exactly the same as before; legal mandates and audit requirements require that much. The casual observer would still see a site evaluation followed by the issuance and discussion of a written report. The same type of site evaluation or inspection will occur, with the sanitarian noting and documenting public health concerns.

The changes will occur in the environment around that function, how sanitarians prepare for and approach the evaluations, how they evaluate the occurrence of noncompliance and how they interact with the client and other site personnel.

Most sanitarians probably have not considered the idea of change interventions, thinking it was included in the site evaluation. In fact, the site evaluation is only the beginning, a needs assessment for the site or the facility. The most significant changes will occur around that evaluation, the environment that supports and allows the intervention to take place. Rather than work entirely on problem discovery and documentation, sanitarians would begin observing attitudes, beliefs and behaviors of the site personnel, to gather data on noncompliant behavior. More time would be allocated to the interviews before and after the site evaluation.

STEP ONE. EXPAND THE EXPLANATION

The first and most significant task is to expand the sanitarian's options regarding environmental noncompliance, to allow he or she to acknowledge other causes of noncompliance and to go back to the holistic, triadic, environmental health paradigm described at the beginning of this book. When faced with noncompliant behavior at a facility or site, sanitarians should have the flexibility of integrating education and consultation with enforcement functions, not turning immediately to discussions of legal consequence. Once the sanitarian begins to explore[195] the possible causes of noncompliance, the intervention design should start to reflect this flexibility. It should no longer be adequate to immediately conclude that enforcement is needed. While this might be true, all options should be explored.

While in theory, that flexibility has always been present through 'professional judgment', knowledge of the true nature of these functions is woefully inadequate. Most public health professionals assume, for instance, that 'education' is a matter of giving the client a pamphlet or newsletter. Some clients, knowledgeable but noncompliant, might take that gesture as insulting. A better approach would be taking the client to the site of a problem, reviewing coping strategies and rehearsing and practicing them with the client. While some clients might rebuff this effort, the mere offer expands the sanitarian's role beyond that of enforcement officer.

The 'education' and 'environment' components of the 'three E's' model (figure 1) can be readily correlated to the behavioral science factors discussed in this book. Since 'education' incorporates information, persuasion and communication, it fits well with problem severity, susceptibility and problem perception in the Model. 'Environment' can correspond to the factors of 'cues to action' 'barriers', 'cost-benefit analysis' and 'perceived self-efficacy'. Acknowledged, this analysis is extremely rough but it reflects the training and mind set sanitarians already have in place, a mind set ready to incorporate behavioral science principles. Sanitarians trained in the environmental health specialties and biological sciences should find this Model and associated concepts familiar and comfortable; it should be a comfortable transition to consider it once more.

The existing mindset of "'enforcement officer", however, is neither comfortable nor comprehensive in a unilateral application. It should never be retired from view, however; clients will attend to the sanitarian's message much better knowing that enforcement is always an option. Nothing in this book implies pampering the client; this is impossible if risks are imminent, and undesirable in any event.

---

[195] This entails actively observing the site or facility, much more than interviewing and asking the client direct questions.

One word, *perceive*, runs through the Model and relevant discussions: sanitarians must begin to actively listen to the client's situation, to understand what factors precipitate or prevent behavioral change. This is not an easy task, requiring patience and skill. The client will not always be amenable, often consumed by the sanitarian's enforcement potential. That is why the process of change will be gradual and will require considerable support from the community and public health administration.

One easy, important change is putting a stronger emphasis on pre- and post-visit interviews. Audit standards already include skeleton versions of both, first for the sanitarian to introduce him or herself and review the facility menus, second to discuss the completed report and legal consequences of noncompliance. These could easily be expanded by only a few minutes to consider the client's state of mind. Other ideas are included below and in the Appendix.

STEP 2. EXPAND SANITARIAN TRAINING OPPORTUNITIES

Once flexibility and individual discretion are built into the intervention design, training is important to assure consistent and accurate use of behavioral science components. We now look at the different subjects where training is needed.

Enforcement

It is ironic, with all of the emphasis on enforcement, that sanitarians often are unaware of legal procedures or how to conduct themselves in a legal setting. More training in legal protocols (Injunctions, warrants, court testimony, depositions, etc.) so that when needed, these processes can be used effectively. Training programs must reflect the concepts discussed under the self-efficacy section so that sanitarians feel capable of completing legal processes; this training should include practice under simulated courtroom or legal scenarios, information from attorneys and judges and practice completing legal documents.

When sanitarians enter a courtroom or attorney's office, they find attorneys are unfamiliar or unimpressed with environmental law. Sanitarians are left to research environmental law, write rough drafts of warrants for the prosecutor and testify in court, all without assistance. If they are called to testify in court, they may not have the aid of the agency counsel unless the agency is named in the case.

Liaison between prosecutors and sanitarians would be an important networking option. Clients must see that when enforcement is used, it is used consistently and strictly, by all sanitarians, with real consequences. Otherwise, they will be glad to extend the process indefinitely, delaying compliance.

Behavioral Health Applications

Sanitarians are well versed in technical and analytical aspects of their work; in order to apply the Model in their work, they need familiarity with behavioral science concepts, particularly as these ideas apply to environmental health activities. All causes of noncompliance must be discussed in conjunction with behavioral science models and concepts. Such aspects would include interviews, training programs, assessing the client's mindset, modeling behaviors, persuasive and communication techniques, and productive use of fear arousal techniques. This training is similar to the existing cultural diversity training, something already provided with most health agencies; in this case, rather than analyzing *cultural* differences, participants would be trained to look for diverse psychological and environmental causes of noncompliance.

Sanitarians might feel uncomfortable adopting a more interactive approach with clients, fearing it might imply weakness or reduced authority. In that sense, the 'interview' could easily turn into an 'interrogation', causing more harm than good. Modeling by trusted and credible staff members (a supervisor or sanitarian trainer) is critical, so that sanitarians understand that these practices are practical and effective. Ongoing training might be needed, for both supervisors and staff, to review persuasive arguments for public health compliance. While no amount of training takes the place of reality, simulation exercises can give practice in interviews, observations, needs assessment, and risk assessment. What is important is the understanding that the process is gradual: all data will not be compiled during one interview or one site visit.

David Mikkola, R.S., M.P.H.

Modify Existing Education Programs

In line with adopting new intervention strategies, education programs, for both sanitarians and the public, must change to emphasize outcome behaviors (including attitude change) rather than merely the mastery of knowledge. At present, trainers emphasize outcomes linked to risk identification and report generation, not to risk communication and abatement.

The training components of knowledge mastery, hazard identification and status documentation, receive the most attention; this training aspect is currently most effective. This type of rote-based training is relatively inexpensive to administer, using a combination of classroom work, learning modules, audiovisual materials, and, to evaluate retention, either an examination or one-to-one interviews.

Instruction in skills mastery and outcome behaviors is a more difficult proposition, however. (Note the contrast in the use of the term *outcome*; in this book, it means long-term risk abatement, *not* risk identification and report generation as current training programs dictate. The latter are only tools to obtain the desired outcome, not ends in themselves.)

It will never be possible to upgrade training programs to provide full skills mastery. Skills modeling and practice can be done in the context of a classroom or learning module, and even to a limited extent in work environments. For example, some client trainers observe participants as they train or monitor conditions under work conditions; sanitarian trainers evaluate sanitarian trainees during actual site inspections. While these are reasonable attempts, it is impractical to approximate completely authentic work conditions, conditions where the evaluator's presence does not skew results. It should also be noted that these efforts still are largely grounded in concept knowledge (risk identification and report generation), not in outcome behaviors (abatement, communication, and intervention). Sanitarians work alone, without the presence of credible role models to reinforce an efficacious work ethic. Required resources for modeling, practicing, and auditing skills would be prohibitive: too much emphasis on reevaluation might be misconstrued as harassment. In addition, resource limits and productivity pressures will restrain the extent of existing evaluation efforts; administrators will always limit these efforts in favor of bringing personnel into productive environments.

Trainers use these limits as an excuse not to extend training efforts; the sanitarian's "professionalism" is used as "evidence" that the individual has received adequate training. This is not a valid excuse, however; that limit occurs in nearly every behavioral change intervention, be it sanitation assessment or the use of the Health Belief Model, and these interventions are still successful. Changes can still occur around these limitations, if training is dynamic, continuous and consistent.

Training Program Design

Having identified flaws in program design, what changes can be made with sanitarian training, staying within the limits of the existing system? Sanitarian trainees receive unending quantities of information; this area, concept mastery, is handled well. While some skills training is included in instruction, this training relates to requirements for audits and matching funds, which stress risk identification and report generation, not risk abatement or communication. (Trainers are content with this definition, believing that the latter concepts [a] cannot realistically be evaluated and [b] they are psychologically influenced, not subject to influence in any event.) This type of instruction, however, carries mastery only to an intermediate phase; while skills are an essential part of the holistic scheme, their impact does not carry over to risk abatement. Skills can be described and modeled vicariously (e.g., audiovisual), but evaluation of skills mastery is an expensive, resource and time dependent task. Supervisory audits and client interviews only approximate the sanitarian's skills mastery. Joint site evaluations are the only effective way to measure the trainee's skills mastery but this is an expensive, resource and time-dependent effort. Reminder forms, such as those in the Appendix, might be cues to action, similar to the impact of reminder postcards[196]. If postcards are used to cue clients toward personal health actions, might cues such as email reminders ('Everyone has been doing a great job submitting those monitoring forms. Keep up the good work!') be used to remind sanitarians?

It is this final phase that matters and must be evaluated. Under the present system, health administrators rely on the sanitarian's

---

[196] Research on postcards as cues to action are numerous; see footnote 162

"professional judgment," presumably developed through academic training, and the hiring process, to assure ultimate skills mastery with risk abatement. These limits have to be acknowledged; sanitarians must have some latitude during site assessments. The extent and reliability of this discretion however, becomes progressively less viable as sanitarians are hired with less extensive and specialized academic training and as restrictive budgets limit the scope of professional audits.

The limits of direct evaluations transfer more emphasis to peripheral methods such as verbal persuasion, vicarious observation, and written documentation (checklists, self-assessments).

The sample forms provided in the Appendix are examples of this type of written feedback; the content would vary with the service program. These tools remind the sanitarian of important concepts from their training and of their commitment to public health. Appendix form number 3 reminds the sanitarian of key *behavioral* science concepts to look for and reinforce during site inspection interviews before and after the evaluation. This form is official and would be attached to the evaluation document. Appendix form number 4 is a reminder checklist for sanitarians to use prior to starting their site evaluations. Appendix form number 5 is a sanitation concern checklist for use by sanitarians to monitor sanitation status and remind them of the most important concepts to evaluate during a site evaluation. All forms are templates for use in any environmental health service program. In this case, they have been completed for use in a food service program. The important point is that some sort of reminder system is used.

There are any number of different varieties of sanitation checklists in existence. The most important thing is that one is used. The sanitarian's task is overwhelming enough without forgetting to check a high-risk sanitation concern. These reminders are critical tools.

The monitoring form would be an intra-office form designed to help sanitarians complete the evaluation; it would not be left with the client. It is an example and would be changed to reflect the various service programs, as well as changing legal standards. There are numerous quality assurance checklists that could be used in its place; most health agencies have one they recommend to clients. This regular written feedback, combined with the existing audit system (review of documents, supervisory site audits), should compensate for the unique, varying nature of the sanitarian's work.

Client education programs

The design of client education programs also must be restructured. As with sanitarian training, these programs more than adequately address knowledge mastery issues; they do *not*, however, address outcome objectives that influence sanitation status and behavioral change. A client might successfully complete an instruction program yet be unable to institute appropriate changes at the facility. While the lecture-examination format is effective at measuring a client's sanitation knowledge, it must be modified to emphasize applications of knowledge toward behavioral change at the facility site, i.e. address outcome expectations, particularly improved sanitation status on-site.

Program design changes would have two parts and require a team-teaching approach. The first portion of the program would remain the same, where information and an examination would determine the client's mastery of the information. This section would, however, describe coping strategies and behavioral objectives using indirect, vicarious modeling. Some limited simulation exercises and modeling would demonstrate skills methodology.

After the client completed knowledge assessment on the examination, the inspecting sanitarian would assist on-site in skills development through employee training programs and written materials (quality assurance checklists, hazard analysis worksheets, HACCP plans, and the like).

STEP 3. DEVELOP NETWORKING STRATEGIES

Networking strategies must be developed to disseminate *consistent and accurate* environmental health information through the community. Networking is an essential component of the triadic evaluation system; it supports the sanitarian's efforts on-site by exposing clients and their support structure to health information in many different venues. As has been mentioned, the existing committee structure used for handling communitywide public health crises might be used for this purpose, albeit on a reduced scale, to meet with representatives of public health concerns (nurses, doctors, hospitals, professional organizations, librarians, government officials, fire and police officials, and school system representatives).

David Mikkola, R.S., M.P.H.

The committee would be used for functions such as public distribution of environmental health pamphlets, newsletters, and recorded media; developing information gathering tools such as surveys and questionnaires; developing communication and marketing campaigns; and developing problem-solving interventions using the information from surveys. On a more basic level, the professionals could learn what their counterparts do, and do not do, within the public health arena. (This comment may sound cynical but it is the sad truth, limiting the ability to function as a team. Bureaucratic delineation of job function promotes ignorance of other job functions.) On a more general level, there would be a significant savings in resources and increases in campaign efficacy.

One main objective would be to assure consistent and accurate delivery of information to all population segments. During the time of year emphasizing food safety, for instance, health educators, nutritionists, doctors, nurses, and sanitarians would all be delivering the same message to food service operators, their families, and significant others.

Another priority would be maintaining a current list of contacts so that public inquiries could be referred quickly and accurately to the most relevant source of information. Perhaps the most important function, however, would be communication between sanitarians and public health stakeholders about their respective concerns and job responsibilities. Otherwise, networking could be a disaster. Historically, the trend among health professionals has been to avoid interaction with the media, for fear they would be misunderstood or misquoted. This reluctance, however, allows inconsistent and inaccurate health information to be distributed by others who are less qualified for that job. It furthers downplays the importance of the sanitarian's profession and position.

Some readers may contend that networking already exists. This is true to some extent. There are communication campaigns and networking for some public health service programs but not environmental health. It is the author's experience that most public health professionals are not aware, familiar with or sympathetic with environmental health services. Further, the communication campaigns and networking in place do not practice the full communication matrix: the emphasis, based on the 'empty vessel' fallacy, is only on disseminating information.

Intra-departmental networking

Within one health agency, health educators, nurses, nutritionists, and sanitarians often misunderstand the nature of their respective service programs. Task delineation models artificially draw bureaucratic lines when there should be intra-agency cooperation. This contributes to ineffective networking, skepticism about other professions and duplication of effort, in the agency and in the community at large. New health employees should spend a day shadowing the other professionals; sanitarians should invite health educators, nurses, and nutritionists to accompany them on an inspection, to offer advice about persuasive and communication aspects. As positive information about each profession disseminates from the agency, **inter**-agency community-wide networking should become more efficient.

Team inspections

Sanitarians will feel additional pressures as the new system is phased into effect. Team inspections are useful tools to relieve these pressures as new skills are learned and mastered. One sanitarian can be sure the report is comprehensive and evaluate, while the second can do interviews, needs assessments, and observations. While administrators may view this as a waste of resources, it actually increases productivity, sanitarian learning, and morale.

STEP 4. SITE INSPECTION EFFICIENCY

As economic conditions decrease the tax base, sanitarians are pressured to complete their work in progressively less time. One site inspection cannot accomplish all requirements of the Model or, for that matter, of the *existing* inspection protocol. While networking will provide some support for the sanitarian's message (clients and their significant others will already have heard that message in other venues), more time will be needed to adequately address the interviews, observations, and needs assessments required by the ideas in this book.

Some time will need to be gained through using risk assessment inspections. More and shorter revisits may be needed. Over the long term, time also will be recouped through fewer enforcement efforts (compliance will be realized through education and consultation efforts).

This scenario suggests a *gradual* implementation of the Model and the realization that the completion of each site inspection depends not on a preset time quota, but on accurate risk assessment and abatement. These tasks will *always* take longer than one site visit to complete. Information gathering will also take longer, as sanitarians must establish a rapport with site personnel and allow lines of communication to develop.

In order to recover inspection time, the emphasis must change. Three phases are essential: *evaluative*, in which facts about risk factors and management attitudes are gathered and organized; *consultative*, in which evaluations are assessed, prioritized, and communicated; and *pre- and post-site evaluation interviews*, in which the purpose of the site evaluation is discussed and later the site report and observations are reviewed.

The evaluative phase is handled well, to the point where it takes too much time during the site visit. This is due to audit standards and the sanitarian's fears of evaluation. The post-site inspection interview occurs, but mainly to obtain the client's signature, not their feedback or questions. In most cases, the pre-site inspection interview does not occur at all. (Sanitarians often are skeptical of any pre-inspection delays for fear the client will make corrections: this skepticism declines with experience, however)

Time could be recovered if risk assessment concepts were actively pursued. Combining one longer comprehensive routine inspection with a shorter risk assessment inspection might recoup time for interviews, assessments, and observations. The risk assessment inspection would emphasize those items with high relative public health risk such as those already noted as critical in the inspection report. Risk assessment would also include reducing inspections in facilities with a smaller risk factor (clients with superior sanitation status could enter into contractual agreements); raising license fees and enforcement protocols for facilities at increased risk; allowing phased compliance programs for low-risk factors (infrastructure, equipment repair[197]); and more

---

[197] Albert Bandura, *Social Foundations of Thought & Action: A Social Cognitive Theory* (New Jersey: Prentice-Hall, 1986)., pp. 161-162, also Albert Bandura, *Social Learning Theory* (Englewood Cliffs: New Jersey, Prentice-Hall, Inc. 1977), p. 83.

basic, incorporating written summaries of sanitation status summaries and management interviews. This might leave more time on the site visit for interviews and consultation. To do this effectively, however, dynamic training will be needed in HACCP ('hazard analysis and critical control points'), quality assurance, and recognition of public health risk. Sanitarians lacking this training might pass over more complicated risk analysis and produce a shorter inspection with low-risk concerns.

This approach differs from the traditional site inspection in several distinct ways: active sanitarian-manager negotiation and communication must be ongoing throughout the site visit[198]; the site visit must be a problem-oriented, risk factor evaluation; and the role of sanitarian as enforcer must evolve into that of facilitator.

---

[198] Vincent Covello and Frederick Allen, "Seven Cardinal Rules of Risk Management," US Environmental Protection Agency, OPA-87-020 4/1988. "Rule 1—Accept and involve the public as a legitimate partner.". Quoted on the Michigan Department of Agriculture website, http://www.michigan.gov/documents.

FINAL SUMMARY

Research shows that exposure to information, as with certified food-service managers,[199] significantly improves attitudes toward sanitarians; networking can support and address the same concerns, both between health professionals and between clients and sanitarians. In addition, the shift from risk identification to risk assessment during inspections can allow more time for interviews and needs assessment. Both networking and site evaluations must be assertive and proactive; causality must be actively sought at each unique site and facility, rather than retrospectively placing each event into a statistically significant slot.

Site evaluations already consider many of the ideas in this book, to one extent or another. The emphasis must change, however, from documentation to risk assessment, and from note-taking to public health impact evaluation. Site inspections must not be confined to a set time period; i.e., inspections and assessments end with abatement of public health risk, *be it in one day or six years*. With this new system, violations are documented within the context of problem analysis, not as an end in themselves.[200] In fact, existing protocols presently allow for repeated site visits; risk assessment studies already advocate the use of longer risk assessment (HACCP-based) inspections once a year.

This discussion does not consider imminent public health hazards, crises in which the client's attitudes, beliefs, and intentions are legitimately irrelevant and a problem must be immediately abated. In those situations, discussions can, and *should* be held with the client *after the fact* to review the situation and recommend changes to avoid any recurrence of the problem. After the situation is under control, the process under discussion can be instituted.

---

[199] Jerry Wright and Lindson Feun, "Food Service Manager Certification: An Evaluation of Its Impact," *National Journal of Environmental Health*, 1986, 49(1): article conclusions p. 15

[200] Food safety regulations have been amended; rather than just two categories, critical and noncritical, there are three risk categories (priority, priority foundation, and core items).

Even acknowledging the importance of education and consultation in a site visit, sanitarians will not have time to incorporate the Model's concepts in one site visit. Research and data gathering alone will take several visits. Organized networking must be a partner in any intervention, emphasizing and supporting information and recommendations introduced during site inspections. Even with regular meetings, correspondence and communication campaigns, it might take some time for sanitarians to see a difference in client attitude and motivation. Public health agencies must be proactive in seeking out contacts in schools, mass media, clinics, hospitals, volunteer agencies, and other health outlets, in the same manner as is presently done for emergency planning coordination services.

In these suggestions, three assumptions are present: (a) sanitarians can only lay the *foundation* for success—networking is essential for long-term success; (b) sanitarians must receive comprehensive training both for purposes of prospective intervention design and for ensuring effective use of legal enforcement tools in short-term acute risk situations; (c) the manager or responsible party on-site must be encouraged to participate in the problem-solving process; and (d) no matter how comprehensive the intervention, some noncompliant behavior will persist and must be expected. It is not the fault of the sanitarian or service program if facility representatives refuse the offer to participate in problem resolution. A sincere offer to negotiate is given; if clients doubt its sincerity or refuse to participate, that is not the sanitarian's fault or concern. Furthermore, such an offer makes subsequent enforcement activities much more credible.

Health educators have researched the Health Belief Model and similar behavioral science concepts for over sixty years; the Model's effectiveness in explaining personal and community-wide public health behaviors has been demonstrated. Research has recently begun in applications to environmental health services such as air pollution mitigation.[201] It is now time for sanitarians to research possible applications of behavioral

---

[201] Robert M. Gray, Josephine M. Kasteler, and Reed H. Geertsen, "Public Attitudes Toward Air Pollution as a Motivational Factor in Taking Action," in *The Annals of Regional Science V. 7 (2)* December 1973 pp. 106-114 (Berlin/Heidelberg: Springer) Abstract cited on link.spinger.com. Only the abstract was referenced to show environmental applications of Health Belief Model)

science concepts to environmental health service programs. The fact that the triadic approach, similar to the Model's structure, has been taught for decades in environmental health and natural science curricula, suggests plausible effectiveness with environmental health service programs.

A natural response is to ask why these explanations of noncompliant behavior must be so complicated. If clients do not understand the message and want the information, why can't they ask for clarification? The answer, according to Rosenstock, might be the "professional distance" between the science-oriented public health practitioner and the client. There is no time to ask questions, questions make clients appear ignorant, and the answers often are loaded with scientific jargon that is difficult to understand.[202]

As with all discussions, time and research will determine the best clarity and statistical fit. This is only the first of many discussions. While models move inquiries in the right direction, time and research will produce the most precise statistical fit. To quote William McGuire,

> Theories provide the confidence and direction for proceeding on a fixed course. Even when the chosen theory is not optimal . . . it suffices to lead us out to some terra cognita with deliberate speed.[203]

---

[202] Irwin M. Rosenstock, PhD, "Patients' Compliance with Health Regimens," *Journal of American Medical Association*, October 27, 1975, 234(4): 402.

[203] William McGuire, "Theoretical Foundations of Campaigns," in Ronald E. Rice and William J. Paisely, eds., *Public Communication Campaigns* (Beverly Hills, London: Sage, 1981), (Beverly Hills, London: Sage, 1981), p. 70.

APPENDIX OF FIGURES

APPENDIX 1
INTERVENTION POINTS IN THE HEALTH BELIEF MODEL

HEALTH BELIEF PHASE	Phase Defined	Strategies
PERCEIVED SUSCEPTIBILITY	Belief about the possibility of getting the condition	Discuss illness case studies (links to current violations), especially those in the vicinity; the wide range of susceptibility to illness and high-risk cases; the individual's personal risk and responsibility (i.e., eating out, preparing food for others); misinformation about food safety revealed during the inspection.
PERCEIVED SEVERITY	Belief about the condition's serious effects	Discuss impact (economic, personal) of condition on individuals, the facility, and the community.
PERCEIVED BENEFITS	Belief that the mandated action will resolve the condition	Review costs and benefits of compliance, eliminating excessive or imagined costs; provide lists of service providers; make complicated actions manageable by separating them into phases.

HEALTH BELIEF PHASE	Phase Defined	Strategies
PERCEIVED BARRIERS	Belief about the costs (economic and otherwise) of the mandated action	Be a resource, model, and educator to the facility and individual; defuse objections to change. If possible, intercede with others (community agencies, facility owners) to help overcome barriers. Be present in the community through networking.
CUES TO ACTION	Pressures (internal and external) to change behaviors	Increase site visits, make community presence known to the facility, and emphasize consistency to all facilities. Reinforce positive progress; bring pressure about relapse and negative actions. Discuss and initiate legal consequences at the first sign of recalcitrance.
PERCEIVED SELF-EFFICACY	Perceived belief in one's ability to take action	Improve and expand available education and training efforts on-site and through networking; model ideal behaviors during site visits, allowing time to practice.

APPENDIX 2
POINTS WHERE SANITARIANS CAN INFLUENCE DECISION MAKING

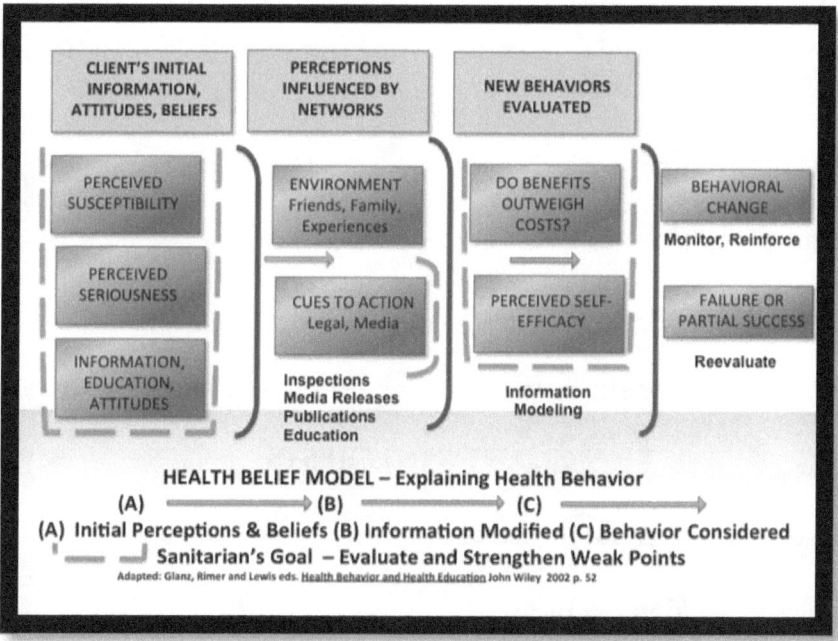

The dashed lines indicate intervention areas; the first and third columns would be addressed during the site visit, the second as part of networking.

APPENDIX 3
EVALUATION INTERVIEWS

(**Instructions:** Use this form to note conversations with site personnel; identify barriers or deterrents to behavioral change (attitudes, beliefs, skills, and resources). Concentrate on high-risk sanitation concerns. *Do not* include confidential or potentially embarrassing information (recipes, finances, personal data).

Date of Interview

Inspection Date/Form No.

Person Interviewed/Sanitarian's Name

===

CLIENT'S INTERESTS

Personal interests, topics useful in future conversations

Topics to avoid in the future

===

FACILITY INFORMATION

Operating Hours (best times for site visits):

Location (how to find the site and gain entry):

Cultural or religious issues (days to avoid a site visit, menu items prepared in a specific manner, language barriers)?

===

CLIENT PERSPECTIVE (Health Belief Model)

Client's Perceptions—Susceptibility, Severity

```
0---------------1---------------2---------------3---------------4---------------5
low (negative)          medium (2.5)            high (positive)
```

Client's Perception of Coping Strategies

```
0---------------1---------------2---------------3---------------4---------------5
low (negative)          medium (2.5)            high (positive)
```

Client's Perception of Barriers

```
0---------------1---------------2---------------3---------------4---------------5
low (negative)          medium (2.5)            high (positive)
```

Client's Perception of Personal Self-Efficacy

```
0---------------1---------------2---------------3---------------4---------------5
low (negative)          medium (2.5)            high (positive)
```

==

Based on this interview, how likely is it that the client will initiate behavioral change (critical items) within the next thirty (30) days ("we know it's difficult to change things overnight. How likely is it that change might start in 30 days?"). Keep the results and evaluate them later.

```
0---------------1---------------2---------------3---------------4---------------5
low (negative)          medium (2.5)            high (positive)
```

Describe positive trends in the facility initiated by the client. (Be certain to find something, however small, even if not related to this report; e.g., new dining room, menu redesigned.) Reinforce those trends with the client.

David Mikkola, R.S., M.P.H.

What areas of the Model need strengthening in order to hasten behavioral change? (Circle)

Attitudes and Beliefs (Susceptibility/Severity)

Barriers to Action

Personal Self-Efficacy (Outcome/Efficacy)

Recommendations for future site visits.

_____

_____

_____

_____

_____

APPENDIX 4
EVALUATION CHECKLIST

Use this checklist to (a) *prepare* for the site evaluation and (b) *remind* yourself of important factors to consider during the evaluation.

Date: ___/___/___

Facility Name & Address: _____

PREPARING FOR THE EVALUATION

In preparing to conduct the site evaluation, have you . . .

(1) **Reviewed the file?** (legal standing, operator's name, high-risk concerns, location, times of operation)

(2) **Assembled the necessary equipment?**
   (a) Flashlight
   (b) Probe thermometer (calibrated)
   (c) Dish machine heat tapes, thermometer
   (d) Sanitizing solution test strips
   (e) Alcohol wipes for probe thermometer
   (f) ens, evaluation forms, notepad, clipboard
   (g) Legal references
   (h) Reference information (legal changes, pamphlets)
   (i) Disposable gloves, head covering
   (j) Computer

In preparing *yourself* for the site evaluation, do you have
   (a) Suitable clothing for the site or activity
   (b) Hair restraints or head covering, hard hat
   (c) Disposable gloves
   (d) Identification badges, business cards

David Mikkola, R.S., M.P.H.

AT THE SITE, BEFORE THE EVALUATION STARTS

(1) Speak with the person in charge
Show your identification, discuss the purpose of your visit, review the menu for high-risk foods or unique processes and invite the manager to accompany you,

Prepare for the evaluation . . . .
Remove outdoor clothing, put on head covering, assemble equipment and wash your hands

DURING THE EVALUATION

(1) Observe employee activities (hand washing, food preparation, food handling)
(2) Check food temperatures, hot and cold
(3) Check storage unit temperatures (refrigerator, freezer, steam table)
(4) Check food temperatures after cooking
(5) Review facility records (employee restriction and exclusion, shellstock tags, records for frozen sashimi fish etc.)
(6) Check food labels, sources, dates
(7) Use a checklist to be sure all concerns are evaluated.

AFTER THE EVALUATION

(1) Discuss the facility's sanitation status with the client, including cited concerns, coping strategies and their expected correction times. Get the client's feedback, including perceived barriers to compliance. Take notes on these concerns for future revisits or for other sanitarians
(2) Discuss positive aspects of the evaluation with the client; if no positive aspects are apparent, ask the client.

APPENDIX 5
SANITARIAN'S CHECKLIST[204]

SANITATION CONCERNS TO OBSERVE
Acceptable (+) Unacceptable (-) or / (not applicable)

Sanitation Concern	+	-	/
General Concerns			
Review compliance with standing orders from previous legal actions or unresolved violations			
Person in charge—demonstrates knowledge			
Pest control—no evidence of pests, integrated pest management, active pest control program,			
Plumbing—no leaks or drippage, cross-connections controlled, approved municipal and on-site supplies			
Exterior refuse controlled and sanitary; pest proof storage; regular collection, clean, covered			
Interior refuse containers covered or emptied			
Highly susceptible population? Review compliance with legal requirements			
Management aware of potential allergens, employees are trained, policy in place			
Changes to facility, equipment or menu that require official review—new foods or food preparation			

---

[204] This template could be used for any environmental health service program: in this case, food service is the example. It is completed with notes from the US Food and Drug Administration 2005 Food Code and should be adapted to include other local issues. Each item should be checked for accuracy before field use; laws are upgraded and vary with each region. Items not addressed could be added at the end of the form.

David Mikkola, R.S., M.P.H.

Review of Menu and Placards			
Foods are accurately and honestly presented			
Consumer advisory language adequate			
Variance, standard operating procedure required? (e.g. smoked/cured foods, reduced oxygen packaging, sous vide, packaged foods for retail sale, cook-chill)—review and evaluate			
Food Source			
Approved source—paperwork, container labels			
Fish served undercooked or raw—proof of blast freezing or procedure to provide the same on site—held 90 days			
Shellfish 'harvest' tags—held 90 days			
Raw animal foods—approved labels, safe handling			
Refrigeration and Freezer Storage			
Food temperatures safe (< 41 degrees F)			
Foods covered/packaged, 6" off floor, not stacked			
Food containers approved			
Ready to eat, potentially hazardous foods dated to hold under 7 days; foods with expired dates discarded			
Foods labeled as to source and content			
Refrigeration and freezer in good repair			
Raw animal foods stored below, away from ready to eat foods			
Raw animal foods stored, by cooking temperature, to protect against contamination			
No drippage, condensation leaks			
Adequate light levels for cleaning			
Graduated thermometers provided at front of unit			
Food Preparation (10-15 minute observation)			
Good employee hygienic practices			

Handling minimized by use of utensils			
Separate utensils and preparation areas for ready-to-eat foods and raw animal foods			
No bare hand contact with ready-to-eat foods			
Alternative policy to bare hand contact—reviewed			
Disposable gloves available where required (sandwiches or salad preparation on menu)			
Gloves changed, hands washed as needed			
Food being prepared protected when not in use			
In-use utensils stored properly			
Limited food supplies under preparation (less than 30 minutes supply)			
Fruits, vegetables washed in approved procedure (approved chemicals if used)			
Safe Preparation Procedures			
'Time as public health control' in use? Signs, procedures, monitoring comply			
Safe thawing procedures—correct process (<70 degree F., circulating water) and limited time period, monitored by employees			
Safe cooling procedures—approved equipment (shallow pans, ice bath, rapid cooling), 2 phase time period (2 hours from 135 degrees F. to below 70 degrees F; under 4 more hours from 70 degrees F. to below 41 degrees F.; temperatures and times monitored by employees			
Safe reheating procedures—proper equipment and time period, temperatures monitored			
Safe food holding temperatures—Hot foods above 135°F. cold foods below 41°F.			
Foods cooked thoroughly (check temperature of food being cooked)			
"long-time, low temperature' foods—processes comply			
Calibrated probe thermometer in use			

Positive Notes: HACCP plan, temperature charts or standard operating procedures in use? Reinforce this positive trend with the client during interviews			
Food Service & Display			
Food on display or in service protected with shields, covers or wrapping			
Served food is not reused but is promptly discarded			
Employee monitor provided			
All you can eat buffet—'new dish' sign provided			
Safe holding temperatures maintained and monitored			
Utensils with extended handles			
Plates, silverware at buffet inverted, protected			
Management is aware of allergen information if needed, has procedure for informing customers			
Employee Personal Hygiene			
Hand washing thorough, as needed			
Hand sinks equipped, convenient, not blocked			
Employees—clean clothes, head coverings and/or hair restraints; clean hands, trimmed fingernails			
No evidence of employee skin infections, illness			
Restriction/exclusion policy in place—employees are aware of policy, records are kept			
Employee health records maintained—as needed, employees are restricted or excluded per policy			
Beverages in approved containers, properly stored			
Approved employee break area provided			
Storage area for personal belongings provided			
Employee changing area			
'No smoking' policy established, enforced—signs provided			

Environmental Health Noncompliance

Equipment and Utensils			
Commercial design and material standards			
Adequate number and capacity to hold food safely			
Good repair, smooth and easily cleanable			
Clean and sanitary in storage, protected, inverted			
Changed regularly in preparation (after use or at least every 4 hours) to avoid cross-contamination			

Cleaning and Sanitizing			
Equipment, utensils cleaned and sanitized at required intervals			
3 step process known and used			
Wash, rinse, sanitize solutions clean			
Chemical or heat sanitizing per standards (tested)			
Chemical test kit present, used			
Warewashing sink, dish machine maintained and clean			
Wiping cloth solutions clean, approved strength, soiled cloths changed or stored properly after use			

Dry Storage			
Approved food containers—labeled			
Approved location not subject to contamination			
Foods 6" off floor on approved shelves OR, if on floor, in moisture-proof, easily movable containers			

Chemicals			
Approved for use in facility; used per directions			
Containers properly labeled			
Chemicals stored safely, to avoid contamination			
Chemicals used safely, to avoid contamination			

David Mikkola, R.S., M.P.H.

Physical Facilities		
Floors, walls, ceilings in good repair		
Lighting adequate and protected		
Ventilation adequate—no excess steam or smoke		
Adequate, convenient restrooms, doors closed		
Outer openings protected, pest proof		

RECOMMENDATIONS:

ADDITIONAL CONCERNS:

FACILITY NAME/ADDRESS
INSPECTING SANITARIAN:
DATE OF INSPECTION:

BIBLIOGRAPHY

American Public Health Association website, http:// www.apha.org/programs/standards/

Ajzen, Icek, and Fishbein, Martin, "Introduction: A Theory of Reasoned Action," *Understanding Attitudes and Predicting Social Behavior* (New Jersey: Prentice-Hall, 1980).

Ajzen, Icek and Fishbein, *Understanding and Predicting Social Behavior* (Englewood Cliffs, New Jersey: Prentice-Hall, Inc. 1980)

Ajzen, Icek, Albarracin, Dolores, and Hornik, Robert, eds., *Prediction and Change of Health Behavior: Applying the Reasoned Action Approach* (New Jersey: Lawrence Erlbaum Associates Publishers, 2007).

Ajzen, Icek, *Attitudes, Personality and Behavior*, 2nd ed. (Berkshire, England, and New York: Open University Press, McGraw-Hill, 2005) (cognitive dissonance, p. 26).

Atkin, Charles K., "Mass Media Information Campaign Effectiveness," in Ronald E. Rice and William J. Paisely, eds., *Public Communication Campaigns* (Beverly Hills: Sage Publications, 1981).

Bandura, Albert, "Self-Efficacy: Toward a Unifying Theory of Behavioral Change," *Psychological Review*, 1977, 84(2): 191-215.

Bandura, Albert, "Self-efficacy Mechanism in Human Agency", *American Psychologist* v. 37 (2) 2/82 pp. 122-147

Bandura, Albert, *Social Foundations of Thought & Action: A Social Cognitive Theory* (New Jersey: Prentice-Hall, 1986).

Bandura, Albert, *Social Learning Theory* (Englewood Cliffs, New Jersey: Prentice-Hall, 1977).

Becker, Marshall, and Maiman, Lois, "Strategies for Enhancing Patient Compliance," *Journal of Community Health*, Winter 1980, 6 (2): 113-133.

Becker, Marshall, PhD, MPH, Kaback, Michael M., MD, Rosenstock, Irwin M., PhD, et al., "Some Influences on Public Participant in a Genetic Screening Program," *Journal of Community Health*, Fall 1975, 1(1): 3-14.

Bloom, Samuel, and Wilson, Robert, "Patient-Practitioner Relationships," in Howard Freeman, et al., *Handbook of Medical*

Sociology, 3rd ed. (Englewood Cliffs, New Jersey: Prentice-Hall, 1963, 1972, 1979), pp. 275-296.

Cartwright, Dorwin, "Some Principles of Mass Persuasion," *Human Relations*, 1949, 2: 253-267.

Community Tool Box website, http://ctb.ku.edu/, Work Group for Community Health and Development at the University of Kansas.

Cook, Charlotte, and Casey, Ralph, "Assessment of a Food-Service Management Sanitation Course," *Journal of Environmental Health*, March/April 1979, 41(5): 281-285.

Covello, Vincent, and Allen, Frederick, "Seven Cardinal Rules of Risk Management," US Environmental Protection Agency, OPA-87-020, April 1988.

California State Journal of Medicine, Unattributed article, October 1922, 20(10): 361. The article states that "the sanitarian, after all, is a more important advance agent for the millennium than the physician."

Dielman, T. E., PhD, Leech, Sharon L., MPH, Becker, Marshall, PhD, MPH et al., "Dimensions of Children's Health Beliefs," *Health Education Quarterly*, Fall 1980, 7(3): 219-238.

Dwore, Richard B., and Matarazzo, Joseph, "The Behavioral Sciences and Health Education: Disciplines with a Compatible Interest?" *Health Education*, May/June 1981: 4-7.

Fishbein, Martin, and Ajzen, Icek, *Belief, Attitude, Intention and Behavior: An Introduction to Theory and Research* (Massachusetts: Addison-Wesley, 1975) (cognitive dissonance, pp. 39-45; fear arousal, pp. 497-508; persuasive communication, pp. 451-509).

http://en.wikipedia.org/wiki/Fear_appeals#The_Extended_Parallel_Process_Model, a discussion of fear drive models and the process of fear arousal.

Fishbein, Martin, and Ajzen, Icek, *Predicting and Changing Behavior: The Reasoned Action Approach* (New York: Psychology Press, 2010).

Feuer, Dale, and Geber, Beverly, "Uh-Oh . . . Second Thoughts about Adult Learning Theory," *Training*, December 1988: 31-32.

Glanz, Karen, Rimer, Barbara K., and Lewis, Frances Marcus, eds., *Health Behavior and Health Education: Theory, Research and Practice*, 3rd ed. (San Francisco: John Wiley & Sons, Jossey-Bass, 2002).

Goldsmith, Francis J., and Hochbaum, Godfrey M., "Changing People's Behavior Toward the Environment," *Public Health Reports*, May-June 1975, 90(3): 231-234.

Gray, Robert M., Kasteler, Josephine M., and Geertsen, H. Reed, "Public Attitudes Toward Air Pollution As a Motivational Factor in Taking Action," *The Annals of Regional Science December, 1973 V. 7* (2) pp. 106-114 (Berlin/Heidelberg: Springer, December 1973). (Abstract cited on link.spinger.com)

Green, Kreuter, et al., *Health Education Planning: A Diagnostic Approach* (California: Johns Hopkins & Mayfield, 1980), pp. 54-55. Discussion of environmental influences on personal health.

Janis, Irving, and Feshbach, Seymour, "Effects on Fear-Arousing Communications," *Journal of Abnormal and Social Psychology*, 1953, 3(48): 78-92.

James, William, "The Sentiment of Rationality," in James, William, *The Will to Believe, Human Immortality* (New York: Dover Publications, 1956), p. 63.

Janz, Nancy, Champion V.L. and Strecher, V. J. "The Health Belief Model," in Glanz, Rimer, and Lewis, eds., *Health Behavior and Health Education: Theory, Research and Practice*, 3rd ed. (San Francisco: John Wiley & Sons, Jossey-Bass, 2002), p. 52 (chart), pp. 45-66 (chapter 3—discussion of Health Belief Model).

Janz, Nancy, and Becker, Marshall, "The Health Belief Model: A Decade Later," *Health Education Quarterly*, Spring 1984, 11(1): 1-47.

Julian, Ernest M., "Certification Programs: Their Effectiveness and Future: A Discussion Paper Prepared for the Second National Conference for Food Protection," unpublished discussion paper, 1984.

Larson, Eric B., Bergman, James, Heidrich, Fred, Alvin, Barbara L., and Scheeweiss, Ronald Eric B. Larson, 'Do Postcard Reminders Improve Influenza Vaccination Compliance?: A Prospective Trial of Different Postcard "Cues"' *Medical Care* V. 20 (6) (June, 1982) pp. 639-648

Lawrence, Lyn, and McLeroy, Kenneth R., "Self-Efficacy and Health Education," *Journal of School Health* October 1986, 56(8): 317-320.

Leavitt, Judith Walzer, "Typhoid Mary: Villain or Victim?" http://www.pbs.org/wgbh/nova/body/typhoid-mary-villain-or-victim.html.

Leventhal, Howard, et al., "The Impact of Communications on the Self-Regulation of Health Beliefs, Decisions and Behavior," *Health Education Quarterly*, Spring 1981.

Leventhal, Howard, "Fear Communications in the Acceptance of Preventive Health Practices," *Bulletin New York Academic Medicine*, November 1965, 41(11): 1144-1161.

Loewenberg, F. M., *Fundamentals of Social Intervention* (New York: Columbia University Press, 1977), p. 193.

Maddux, James E., and Rogers, Ronald W., "Protection Motivation and Self-Efficacy: A Revised Theory of Fear Appeals and Attitude Change," *Journal of Experimental Social Psychology*, September 1983, 19(5): 469-479.

McGuire, William J., "Theoretical Foundations of Campaigns", in *Public Communication Campaigns*, Rice, Ronald E. and Paisley, William J. eds. (Beverly Hills, London: Sage, 1981) pp. 41-70

McGuire, William J., "Behavioral Medicine, Public Health and Communication Theories," *Health Education*, May/June 1981: 8-13.

Penning, Harold K., and Rodman, Vay A., "'Food Service Managerial Certification: How Effective Has It Been?" *Dairy and Food Sanitation*, July 1984, 4(7): 260-264.

Petty, Richard, and Cacioppo, John, *Attitudes and Persuasion: Classic and Contemporary Approaches* (Iowa: Wm. C. Brown, 1981).

Petty, Richard, and Cacioppo, John, *Communication and Persuasion: Central and Peripheral Routes to Attitude Change*, in *Springer Series in Social Psychology* (New York: Springer-Verlag, 1986).

Polgar, Steven, "Health and Human Behavior: Areas of Interest Common to the Social and Medical Sciences," *Current Anthropology* April 1962, 3(2): 159-205.

Ray, Michael, and Wilkie, William, "Fear: The Potential of an Appeal Neglected by Marketing,"' *Journal of Marketing*, 1970, 34(1): 54-62.

Rice, Ronald E., and Paisley, William J. eds, *Public Communication Campaigns* (Beverly Hills: Sage Publications, 1981).

Rich, Ben R. *Clarence Leonard (Kelly) Johnson: 1910-1990 A Memoir* (Washington, DC: National Academies Press, 1995)

Rosenberg, Jennifer, "Typhoid Mary: The Sad Story of a Woman Responsible for Several Typhoid Outbreaks," website www.history1900s.about.com.

Rosenstock, Irwin M., PhD, "Historical Origins of the Health Belief Model," in Becker, Marshall H. Ph.D., M.P.H. editor, *The Health Belief Model and Personal Health Behavior* (Thorofare, New Jersey: Charles B. Slack, Inc. 1974) [reprint of *Health Education Monograph*

1974 (2)], pp. 1-8. Early presentations of the Model emphasize that "it is the world of the perceiver that determines what he will do and not the physical environment . . ." Environmental influences on perception were acknowledged later.

Rosenstock, Irwin M., PhD, "Patient's Compliance with Health Regimens," *Journal of the American Medical Association*, October 27, 1975, 234(4): 402-403.

Rosenstock, Irwin, "The Health Belief Model and Preventative Health Behavior," in Becker, Marshall H. Ph.D., M.P.H. editor, *The Health Belief Model and Personal Health Behavior* (Thorofare, New Jersey: Charles B. Slack, Inc. 1974) [reprint of *Health Education Monograph* 1974 (2)], pp. 27-59

Rosenstock, Irwin M., Strecher, Victor, and Becker, Marshall, "Social Learning Theory and the Health Belief Model," in *Health Education Quarterly*, 1988, 15(2): 175-183.

Shattuck, Lemuel, *Report of the Sanitary Commission of the State of Massachusetts—1850* (http://wwwdeltaomega.org/shattuck.pdf). The report suggests a generalized profession of "sanitarian" that would share attributes of several professions in order to address different varied public health concerns.

Soames Job Ph.D., R. F., "Effective and Ineffective Use of Fear in Health Promotion Campaigns," *American Journal of Public Health*, February 1988, 78(2): 163-167.

Sutton, Stephen, "Fear-Arousing Communications: A Critical Examination of Theory and Research," *Social Psychology and Behavioral Medicine*, 1982, pp. 303-325.

UCLA Department of Epidemiology, "Who is John Snow?" Books, biographies, images about John Snow. See http://www.ph.ucla.edu/ei/snow.html

US Centers for Disease Control, *Morbidity and Mortality Weekly Report*, 58(22): 609-615.

US Government, Health and Human Services, Office of Disease Prevention and Health Promotion, "Vision: Healthy People in Health Communities-Mission: Promote Physical and Mental Health and Prevent Disease, Injury, and Disability," November 28, 2000, Public Health Functions Project.

World Health Organization website http://www.who.int/topics/environmental_health/en/.

Wright, Jerry, and Feun, Lindson, "Food Service Manager Certification: An Evaluation of Its Impact," *National Journal of Environmental Health*, 1986, 49(1): 12-15.

Yiannis, Frank, *Food Safety Culture: Creating a Behavior-based Food Safety Management System* (New York: Springer Publications 2009) Abstract taken from the book description on Amazon.com web site as an example of behavioral science applications to environmental health.

Zander, Alvin, "Influence People in the Face to Face Setting: Research Findings and Their Application," unpublished paper presented to the Society of Public Health Educators on November 11, 1961.

Zemke, Ron, and Zemke, Susan, "Thirty Things We Know for Sure about Adult Learning," *Training* July, 1988: 57-61.

ABOUT THE AUTHOR

David Mikkola is a registered sanitarian in the state of Michigan. He worked for thirty-one years for two Michigan public health departments, primarily inspecting restaurants and swimming pools but also working in environmental health education. He spent twenty-five years teaching public education programs in food sanitation and swimming pool sanitation. His education includes a bachelor of arts degree in secondary school education, a bachelor of science degree in environmental health, and a masters degree in public health with a concentration in health education.

It was during his graduate studies that he became interested in alternative explanations for environmental noncompliance—why people do not accept the sanitarian's inspection results in spite of legal enforcement. The inspection system in use appeared to resort too quickly to the use of enforcement measures when some clients seemed amenable to education and persuasion. Health behavior concepts and models supported the need for a new approach. From this interest evolved this book about a new system for conducting environmental assessments, a new explanation for noncompliance. David currently works as an environmental consultant and lives in southeastern Michigan.

ABOUT THE BOOK

Sanitarians often wonder about the effectiveness of their site evaluations—whether or not the client listens and why noncompliance persists. Their academic training emphasizes a three-pronged approach (education, consultation, and enforcement) toward the analysis and abatement of sanitation concerns; any number of social, political and economic factors, however, deemphasize this approach, stressing the use of legal means to gain compliance. While enforcement and legal actions tend to produce short-term compliance, a roller-coaster effect often results in the long term recurrence of noncompliance. Why? This book analyzes the reasons, looking at ways to integrate health behavior models with the existing inspection based system to design more effective intervention strategies. Education, consultation, and enforcement are melded to produce a more comprehensive approach to site evaluations. Community networking is advanced as an important support system often underutilized by health agencies. In the process, sanitarians are offered suggestions for using these ideas during their site visits.

www.ingramcontent.com/pod-product-compliance
Lightning Source LLC
Chambersburg PA
CBHW032022170526
45157CB00002B/815